Successful Breastfeeding

A PRACTICAL GUIDE FOR NURSING MOTHERS

Successful Breastfeeding

by Nancy Dana and Anne Price

Illustrations by Patricia Carey

Photography by Sue Silker
Glen Silker Studios

ⅢMeadowbrook
Distributed by Simon and Schuster
New York

Library of Congress Cataloging in Publication Data

Dana, Nancy.
   Successful breastfeeding.

   Bibliography: p. 1. Breast feeding. I. Price, Anne.
II. Title. RJ216.P698   1985   649'.33   85-13611
ISBN 0-88166-018-3 (pbk.)
ISBN 0-671-55611-8 (Simon & Schuster: pbk.)

Published by Meadowbrook, Inc., Deephaven, MN
BOOK TRADE DISTRIBUTION by Simon and Schuster, a division of
Simon & Schuster, Inc., 1230 Avenue of the Americas,
New York, NY 10020
ISBN 0-88166-018-3
S&S Ordering Number 0-671-55611-8
85 86 87 10 9 8 7 6 5 4 3 2 1
Printed in the United States of America.

Authors: Nancy Dana and Anne Price
Managing Editors: Thomas Grady and Margery Hughes
Art Direction: Nancy MacLean
Design: Mary Foster
Keyline: Mike Tuminelly
Production: Wendy Lentsch
Photography: Glen Silker Studios
Illustrations: Patricia Carey
Clothing: Courtesy of Maternal Instincts

The authors, editors, reviewers and publisher disclaim all responsibility arising from any adverse effects or results that occur or might
occur as a result of the inappropriate application of any of the
information contained in this book. If you have a question or
concern about the appropriateness or application of the techniques
described in this book, consult your health-care professional.

Contents

Dedication   This book is lovingly dedicated to

Neal,

for your endless love,
support and understanding.

Love, Anne

Tad and Tucker,

for your sweet
pride and enthusiasm.

Love, Mom

Acknowledgments

Our special thanks to

Our models . . . Sarah, Randal and Christopher Barnes; Susan, Kira and Bryn Bundlie; Lisa, Armando, Analisa and Cristina Calderon; Barbara and Laura Gabatino; Mary, Andrea and Daniel Hartman; Shirley Kelly; Anne and Maggie McQuillan; Kathy Monsoor; Diane and Rosemary Schlosser; Duane Simms; Joan and Bob Spence; Barbara and Emily Stigall; Stacie and Carson Young.

Marnie Henderson, Mary Gerhardt and Jackie Frazier, for your careful evaluation of our manuscript. We appreciate the time and effort that you spent, and your objective comments helped us give this book its final form.

Georgann Marx, for the time and care you gave to the valuable exercise program you developed for us. But most of all, thanks for your generosity and patience with our endless questions and requests for your time and knowledge.

Marion Galant, Debra Schwartz, Shira Salzberg, Connie Ellefson, Michele Scheer, Mary Grady and Dana Paris, for your lovely, personal expressions about your own breastfeeding relationships. They are a beautiful addition to our book.

Lev, Mikki and Gabriel, for your love for me and your acceptance of my spending the time it took to write this book.

Thomas Grady, our editor. We appreciate your patience and perseverance and your acceptance of our philosophies and expectations for this book. Your guidance has been enlightening and invaluable.

Maggie Hughes, our editor. We never would have successfully pulled together all those final details without your superior organizational skills. Our bonus was in finding organizer, editor and friend all in one package.

Introduction

Breastfeeding your baby is one of the most loving and natural experiences you will ever have. During recent years, breastfeeding books have convinced more and more mothers to breastfeed. These women have found that breastfeeding, although natural, is not always problem-free. SUCCESSFUL BREASTFEEDING takes up where other books on the subject leave off. We offer you the facts, practical advice and up-to-date techniques you need to succeed.

Elements that contribute to a satisfying experience are emphasized. For example you will find:

• five basic principles for successful breastfeeding

• a guide to preventing and solving the most common breastfeeding difficulties

• new exercises to prevent or relieve a nursing backache

• a guide to food and nutrition for the first year of your baby's life

• personal accounts of breastfeeding mothers

A "successful breastfeeding" experience means something different to each breastfeeding mother. SUCCESSFUL BREASTFEEDING will give you the tools to breastfeed successfully on your own terms and will offer you more thorough factual information than is presented in other breastfeeding books. The easy-to-read format and step-by-step illustrations and photos are designed to make the information accessible and usable to you.

Realizing the social and family implications of breastfeeding, we also provide helpful strategies for:

• involving siblings and fathers

• dealing with physical, psychological and social obstacles

• choosing a weaning philosophy

The majority of women today are making the choice to breastfeed their new babies. Those who are most successful are those armed with the knowledge they need.

Whether you are a new or an experienced mother, if you have chosen to breastfeed, SUCCESSFUL BREASTFEEDING can guide you through your nursing experience, provide the confidence you need to overcome difficulties, and give the skills you need to achieve a comfortable and satisfying nursing relationship.

Chapter One The Advantages of Breastfeeding

A s a prospective parent, you are no doubt looking eagerly to the future, preparing for the arrival of your new baby. Your life seems filled with questions. Which crib shall we buy? What color shall we paint the baby's room? Where shall we have the baby? What shall we name the baby? Shall we breastfeed or bottlefeed?

Your mother bottlefed. Your best friend breastfed. Your neighbor did some of each. You have been sifting through the stories from all sides and are trying to make the best decision for you.

If You Have Already Decided To Breastfeed

Many of you have already decided to breastfeed your new baby and feel committed to that choice. Be assured that you have made the best choice and that you have a warm and rewarding experience ahead of you.

If You Have Not Yet Decided To Breastfeed

Perhaps you have not yet decided; you have heard stories of women who could not, or did not want to breastfeed, and you are not sure of your chances for success. We want to take a moment to refute the most commonly cited arguments for not breastfeeding.

Ten Myths About Breastfeeding

The Myth	*The Fact*
1. Breastfeeding will tie you down.	A breastfed baby is so portable that she can go anywhere you do with ease. There are no bottles to prepare, nor will you ever be unprepared to feed her. And if you do have to be away from your baby, it is easy to leave expressed milk for her until you return.
2. Breastfeeding ruins the shape of your breasts.	Your breasts enlarge during pregnancy and fill with milk after the birth, whether or not you are going to breastfeed. If damage is done, it takes place independent of your plans to nurse your baby.
3. Breastfeeding is too much bother.	Breastfeeding is far less bother than preparing and feeding bottles, especially in the middle of the night.
4. Breastfeeding will hurt.	Breastfeeding does not hurt, even if your baby has teeth, because her tongue protrudes over her bottom gums when she nurses.
5. Breastfeeding is impossible if you do not have enough milk.	Your body operates upon a supply-and-demand system that allows your baby to increase or decrease your supply to meet her needs.
6. Breastfeeding is impossible if your breasts are too small (or too large).	Breast size is determined by fatty tissue and in no way affects your ability to nurse, since the number of milk ducts in your breasts is the same, no matter what size they are.
7. Breastfeeding leaves the father feeling left out.	Fathers of breastfed babies feel proud and supportive of breastfeeding, and they find many warm and special ways

8. Breastfeeding makes it hard to lose weight.

On the contrary, breastfeeding burns calories because of what goes to your baby in your milk and the energy spent producing it.

9. Breastfeeding requires a very restricted diet.

Most breastfeeding mothers do not change the types of food they eat at all.

10. Breastfeeding is impossible if you are going back to work.

Many mothers continue to nurse very successfully after returning to work. Working and nursing need not be mutually exclusive.

In reality, breastfeeding is a simple, wonderful act, and we know that you can breastfeed successfully. On the following pages we will describe the many advantages of breast milk for the baby and explain the advantages of breastfeeding for both the mother and child.

Advantages of Breastfeeding

For Mom

Weight loss is more easily achieved after your baby's birth.

Fewer menstrual cycles are experienced because of hormonal changes that occur with lactation.

Beneficial hormone release helps your uterus return to pre-pregnancy size.

Breastfeeding serves as a tranquilizer for you, and it contributes to the warm feelings that surround caring for your child.

It is convenient to breastfeed. Just pull up your blouse and

For Baby

The act of breastfeeding naturally satisfies the vital need of your baby to suck.

Neurological stimulation starts earliest with a breastfed baby.

Breastfeeding advocates believe that breastfed babies are less prone to dental caries.

Breastfeeding provides your baby with significant protection against allergies.

Breastfed babies have seven times fewer the number of infections than do bottlefed babies.

the meal is ready—sterile, warm and pre-mixed.

Breastfeeding promotes frequent contact with your baby, and it can play an important part in the bonding process.

Breast milk offers a financial savings since it is free.

Breastfeeding provides antibodies which help to halt bacterial growth.

Breastfeeding provides every nutrient your baby needs for brain growth and good overall physical development.

Breast milk is easy for your baby to digest, which results in more efficient use of the milk.

Advantages of Breast Milk—A Living, Life-Giving Fluid

Colostrum The first fluid present in the breasts in late pregnancy and in the first postpartum days is colostrum, a thick, yellowish substance that is gradually replaced as a mother's milk "comes in." Although colostrum is present for only a short time and in small quantities, it is highly valuable to your newborn. Here are some reasons why.

Nutrition. Colostrum, which is quite different from mature breast milk, meets a newborn's specific needs by providing much higher concentrations of the fat-soluble vitamins, a higher mineral content and many more white blood cells than mature breast milk. Its protein content is many times greater than that of breast milk, offering the infant nourishment that keeps her blood sugar level up and provides her with energy. Colostrum's comparatively low fat content is also ideal, since an infant's system is much less capable of digesting fat in the early days. The fluid content is also very low, but babies are born with a fluid reserve that lasts until your milk comes in.

Antibodies. Colostrum contains vast stores of antibodies that protect the infant from both viral and bacterial infections. They virtually cleanse the intestinal tract of infections and organisms, and continue to protect the baby well beyond the age of six to twelve weeks when she begins to produce her own antibodies.

Laxative. Colostrum has a significant laxative effect on a newborn. The stool that accumulates in utero is a thick, sticky substance called *meconium,* which contains a great amount of bilirubin (cast-off excess red blood cells associated with jaundice, see page 118). Bilirubin can be reabsorbed from the intestines into the bloodstream if the meconium is not excreted soon after birth. Colostrum's laxative effect clears out the meconium, discourages jaundice, and prepares the intestinal tract for its new postpartum functions.

Allergy prevention. The intestinal walls of a newborn are quite permeable, so they allow bilirubin, infectious organisms, and even whole, undigested food proteins to pass through into the bloodstream. Many authorities believe that colostrum protects a breastfed baby from allergy through a process called "gut closure." If this process does not occur, the whole proteins that pass into the bloodstream can cause the baby to become sensitized to that particular protein (for example, soy or cow's milk). This is a major way food allergies can develop in a baby.

Nutritional Content of Breast Milk

Because breast milk is specifically designed for the human species, it is perfect for human development. Although infant formulas can come relatively close to imitating human milk, they can never completely duplicate breast milk.

While there are many different kinds of formula, most use cow's milk as their base. But since calves have growth requirements far different from those of infants, their milk is not really suitable for babies. (Though opinion fluctuates, many medical professionals do not recommend giving cow's milk to infants under one year of age.) Formula manufacturers have tried to compensate for these differences by diluting cow's milk to lower the amount of protein per ounce and by adding vitamins and minerals.

Below we will look at the basic nutritional components of breast milk to see how our milk meets the needs of our babies most perfectly. Since cow's milk is the basis of most infant formulas, we will offer comparisons between it and human breast milk.

Protein. Human milk has about half the protein of cow's milk, one effect of which is to increase the number of necessary nursings in a day. This gives lots of contact for both the mental stimulation and the emotional development that babies need.

The composition of the protein in breast milk is also different from the composition of protein in cow's milk. Amino acids, the building blocks of protein, are arranged in human milk so that about 90 percent of the protein in breast milk (more than in any other food) is usable by the infant.

Fat. The fat content of human milk is only slightly higher than that of cow's milk, but since cow's milk is diluted to reduce the protein, so the amount of fat, too, is now reduced to a level below breast milk. This in turn reduces the amount of fat-soluble vitamins present. The ratio of saturated to unsaturated fats is also very different in human milk. Finally, the composition of the fats in breast milk makes more calcium available for the growth of strong bones and teeth.

Carbohydrates. Breast milk contains about 50 percent more of its primary carbohydrate, lactose, than cow's milk. Lactose provides energy and produces an acidic environment in the intestines that discourages bacterial growth. It is used by the baby at an even pace, whereas the sucrose found in many formulas is dispersed too rapidly, causing highs and lows in the infant's blood sugar level.

Water and Salts. There is more water in breast milk than in formula or cow's milk, so a breastfed baby needs no water supplement, unlike her bottlefed counterpart. Cow's milk also has a much higher concentration of salts, like sodium, chloride and potassium, so a baby drinking cow's milk in any form needs lots of water to help her tiny kidneys wash these extra salts out of her system. In contrast, the level of salts in breast milk is quite low, so a baby can use them quite effectively.

Vitamins and Minerals. As with all the other components in breast milk, the vitamin and mineral content is faultless. As modern scientists began to study breast milk, they often thought they had found a deficiency, as in vitamin D, for instance. Researchers could not find this fat-soluble vitamin in the fat portion of breast milk. Further research finally noted a new type of vitamin D in the water portion. Some elements, like calcium, seem to be present in rather low amounts, but a baby's system uses the calcium that is there very efficiently. By contrast, the mineral content in cow's milk and in formulas is far too high for an infant, and it places a great strain on the baby's kidneys.

Iron. A baby is born with sufficient iron stores to last at least until six months of age. Although breast milk is low in iron, cow's milk is even lower, and what little iron there is in breast milk is used with about 50 percent efficiency, while the iron found in cow's milk preparations has less than a 10 percent absorption rate. Because of these differences, a breastfed baby has no need for the iron supplement that is often given to a bottlefed baby. In fact, since bacteria needs iron for growth, too much iron in her intestines could make her more prone to bacterial illness. (See Lactoferrin, page 10.)

Digestibility of Breast Milk

Since human milk is perfectly suited to an infant, it is far more easily digested by the newborn than any other substance, resulting in a number of advantages or effects. Cow's milk formula, whose proteins form large, tough curds in the stomach, is much more difficult to digest.

• The proteins in breast milk are primarily the whey type, as opposed to the predominantly casein-type proteins found in cow's milk and infant formula. When an infant digests whey proteins, the very small, soft curds that form do not strain her tiny digestive system. Her system can extract every morsel of nutrition from a food that is so easily digested.

• Because this food is so readily assimilated by the infant, it takes only about an hour and a half for her system to digest a feeding thoroughly, so breastfed babies tend to eat more frequently than do their formula-fed friends.

• Because breast milk is so efficiently used and because of its composition, the stools of a breastfed baby are often quite soft, runny and yellowish in color. Soft stools are ideal since they do not stress a baby's elimination system. Constipation, which can agonize a mother and baby, is rarely a problem for a breastfed baby, although a new mother may suspect it when her baby seems to strain and grunt when passing a stool. This rather dramatic effort is natural and is not an indication of hard stools.

• Breast milk (even when spit up) and a breast milk stool have a sweet, clean scent, an advantage that is not very significant in health terms, but vastly appreciated in day-to-day life with a new baby.

Breast Milk and Brain Growth

It has been said that the human fetus actually needs eighteen months to develop, but since it grows too large for a mother to carry in utero after nine months, it finishes its development outside the womb. This seems especially true of the growth of the brain, which proceeds at a remarkable rate in the early months after birth. When a baby is perfectly nourished, every nutrient that is needed for brain growth will be available.

• **Lactose,** the sugar that is present only in milk and is an element essential to brain growth, is found in greater quantities in breast milk than in cow's milk. It supplies energy to allow the rapid brain growth to take place, and when it is digested, it produces galactose, a component crucial to the coating of nerve fibers.

• **Taurine,** an amino acid that new research indicates is an important element for brain growth, is almost nonexistent in cow's milk, and a new baby cannot manufacture it. However, it is abundant in human breast milk.

Protection from Infection

When we see the many complex and interrelated ways that breast milk protects our babies from infection, it is easy to believe the statistics that tell us that breastfed babies have one-seventh the number of infections that bottlefed babies have.

• **Antibodies** are proteins that neutralize disease-causing microorganisms. While a baby receives some antibodies in utero, such as Immunoglobulin G (and it was once thought that this was the extent of protection a mother provided for her baby), we now know that more antibodies are present in colostrum and breast milk. The breast itself also performs a miraculous function that is not yet clearly understood. When a breastfed baby is exposed to a germ, so is the mother's breast and it begins to manufacture an antibody to the germ, even if that organism is not present in the mother. After being manufactured in the breast, this antibody is passed through the breast milk to the baby.

• A vital antibody, **secretory IgA,** operates differently in a baby's system than do the other antibodies. Most antibodies travel through the bloodstream, but a secretory immunoglobulin goes directly to the site (the intestine, for instance) of the offending organism and begins to work. Since many potentially troublesome organisms are first found in mucous areas like the throat or in the intestinal tract, the ability of secretory IgA to work "on site" makes it possible to halt bacterial growth quickly.

• **Lactoferrin,** a protein in breast milk that aids the immune system, is iron-binding, so it gobbles up iron that harmful bacteria might otherwise use for growth. (See Iron, above.)

• **Other proteins** in breast milk also fight against infection. For example, the enzyme lysozyme is primarily an anti-infective, as opposed to nutritive, protein.

• The **sugars** in breast milk produce an acidic environment in the intestinal tract that helps prevent the growth of disease-causing bacteria. When the intestine is appropriately acidic, normal healthy bacteria can flourish, and harmful bacteria cannot.

• The **interferon** that breast milk manufactures helps a baby in still another way to defend herself against infection. The white blood cells in breast milk, which closely resemble those in blood, operate by reacting to a virus in the system: they produce interferon, which works to warn surrounding cells of the approaching danger.

Breast Milk and Weight Gain

A baby's weight always seems to be a source of concern to a new mother, even though a totally breastfed baby is going to gain weight at an appropriate rate. Some understanding of what appropriate gain really is, and why we all have such specific expectations about it, can alleviate your concern.

Our expectations about how much weight our babies should gain usually begin with those little growth charts that are plotted for us by medical professionals. But since many of these charts are based on the "average" growth of bottlefed babies, they do not reflect the normal growth that nature intended from breast milk. A breastfed baby's growth will be different from that of a formula-fed infant.

If your baby seems to fall at either the very low or very high end of the scale, rest assured that if she is totally breastfed and seems healthy and happy, her gain is probably appropriate for her as an individual. Breastfeeding will ensure that your baby will reach her genetic potential, which may be lighter or heavier than the "average."

One difference in weight gain is the result of differences between feeding systems. Since a breastfeeding mother does not measure the amount of milk she gives her baby, there is not a temptation to coax down every last ounce, as there is with bottlefed babies. A breastfed baby is free to take only as much as her hunger tells her she needs at each feeding. Eating only to satisfy true hunger is far less likely to produce obese adults.

Cholesterol

Everyone knows the risks associated with high levels of cholesterol in the blood of adults, so there is concern about the very high level of cholesterol in breast milk. For a baby, however, cholesterol is a necessary form of fat that helps develop the nervous system. It now seems that the very high level of cholesterol in breast milk serves to teach the baby's system how to metabolize it. Preliminary evidence indicates that we may discover that breastfed babies grow up to be capable of metabolizing cholesterol. This will result in lower levels of cholesterol in their blood so they will have less risk of developing circulatory diseases associated with cholesterol.

Protection from Allergies

Breastfeeding helps to prevent allergies. While some babies are allergic, or very sensitive, to a food in the mother's diet (most commonly cow's milk and dairy products), the baby is *not* allergic to the breast milk, only to the foods that went into it. If the mother eliminates or cuts down her intake of that offending food or food group, the baby's symptoms will go away and breastfeeding can continue quite nicely.

Statistics show clearly that breastfeeding provides significant protection, especially to anyone with a family history of allergy. One study of well over one thousand babies shows that the longer a baby is breastfed, the lower the chance that she will become allergic.

Duration of Breastfeeding	With Family History of Allergy	With No Family History of Allergy
4 days	7.5 percent	4.1 percent
1-2 months	7.3 percent	2.4 percent
6 months and up	4.0 percent	0.0 percent

The major protection from allergy is provided by the process of gut closure (described earlier), through which a baby's intestinal walls are made impermeable to whole proteins. A baby's chances for being allergic are statistically reduced even if she is fed colostrum for only a few days.

Very often, the younger the baby, the worse the allergy. That is why we often hear that a baby has outgrown an allergy. It follows, then, that the older a baby is before being introduced to a possible allergen, the better her chances are of being able to handle it. A bottlefed baby with an allergic predisposition to cow's milk will react violently when it is introduced in infancy and may retain that allergy throughout her life. However, if that same baby were breastfed and received no cow's milk until after the age of twelve months, she may well be able to tolerate it at an older age.

Fewer Dental Caries

It was once thought that breastfeeding caused an increase in dental caries (tooth decay), but this has been shown to be incorrect. Although, a breastfed baby is far less prone to dental caries. The way a baby nurses at the breast is part of the reason. When a baby nurses, she pulls the nipple far back into her mouth and draws out the milk by the reflexive action of suck-and-swallow. Therefore, the milk comes into contact with only a small portion of the back of her mouth (not her teeth) and it is immediately and reflexively swallowed. A bottle, however, does not reach as far into the baby's mouth, and milk can easily leak out of the nipple and come in contact with her teeth.

Night nursings in bed rarely contribute to tooth decay. It used to be thought that a baby's mouth was coated with breast milk virtually all night long. But when a baby nurses during the night, she can really get milk only when she is actively nursing on the breast. As soon as she dozes off again, milk no longer flows from the breast, and the nipple usually slips out of her mouth entirely.

Financial Savings

An avid breastfeeding mother will often claim that one of the advantages of breastfeeding is a significant financial savings, since breastfeeding is free. Although this is not quite true, it is closer to the truth than the claim that a breastfeeding mother eats so much more in order to produce milk, she saves nothing.

In reality, a breastfeeding mother does have additional nutritional and caloric needs, but they are not so great as some might think. An additional 500 calories a day will make up for the calories spent producing milk, and those calories do not need to come from steak or caviar. It would cost (at this writing) about $1.50 a day *more* to bottlefeed than it would to breastfeed, a savings of about $250.00 in six months, roughly the cost of a major appliance.

Breast Milk Is Constantly Changing

One fascinating aspect of breast milk that can never be duplicated is its ability to change. For a period of time between colostrum and mature milk, for instance, there is a fluid called transitional milk that is a mix of the last of the colostrum and the first of the breast milk. In this way the baby is gradually "weaned" from colostrum to breast milk. It may be nature's way of giving the baby a chance to adjust to a new taste.

Mature milk also varies from the beginning to the end of each feeding. The milk a baby receives in the early part of the feeding, called foremilk, is rather thin and watery, but it contains most of the nutrients. Hindmilk, which is present at the end of the feeding, is higher in fat and calories. Allowing the baby to nurse until she is finished will afford her the value of receiving her full complement of both foremilk and hindmilk.

Also, since a woman's supply begins to diminish when her baby begins to wean, the protein content rises, so that in actuality the baby weans at a slower rate.

Advantages of the Act of Breastfeeding

To the Baby
Development of Teeth, Jaw and Mouth

The vigorous work that a baby must do to draw milk from the breast contributes to and enhances her facial development. When a baby drinks from a bottle she must try to make her mouth fit around the nipple, whatever its shape. But a mother's nipple readily shapes itself to the baby's mouth, and the baby uses entirely different muscles to milk the breast. This difference, combined with the vigorous work required, causes the baby's jaw, teeth and mouth to develop optimally. She will be far less likely to develop any malformation of the teeth, jaw or palate.

Natural Urge to Suck

A baby is born with a naturally strong urge to suck, which is probably nature's way of ensuring that she nurses enough to get sufficient nourishment and loving contact. Because the mother's breast conforms to the shape of her baby's mouth and because nursing provides closeness with the mother, time at the breast is the optimal way to satisfy this vital need. The need for sucking is as urgent and vital a need as any to the baby and she will not let it go unsatisfied. Some babies seem to have a greater need for sucking than others, and some probably just enjoy it more than others. In any case, it is not a need to be overlooked.

Neurological Benefits

A crucial part of the neonatal development of a child is the progression of two-sided activities. This right and left orientation (as in crawling) seems to prepare an infant for more complex tasks like reading. The stimulation of the two sides seems to start earliest if the baby is breastfed. As she nurses, her eyes naturally search out the face of her mother, who nurses her alternately on the right and left breast. The baby thus must train her eyes to find her mother's face from either side. Although a bottlefeeding mother may occasionally switch sides, she is much more likely to feed her baby only on the side that is more comfortable for her, since there is no compelling reason to alternate.

To the Mother
Weight Loss

During your pregnancy, your weight may increase by twenty-five to thirty-five pounds, a gain that is made up of baby, amniotic fluid, stores of water, nutrients and fat to prepare you to breastfeed. If you do not breastfeed, however, it will be much harder to lose the weight your body has stored fo that purpose. Here is why.

When you are breastfeeding, you will use from 600 to 800 calories a day for the milk itself and the energy it takes to produce it. If you follow the usual dietary recommendations, you will eat about 500 extra calories a day because of your increased hunger; the additional 200 to 300 calories will come from the stores built up in pregnancy. Were you not breastfeeding, you would have to eliminate that many calories from your diet in order to lose weight as fast.

This formula, of course, cannot possibly apply to all women in all circumstances. It is more difficult for some women, breastfeeding or not, to lose weight than for others. While you may have a bottlefeeding friend who loses weight more rapidly than you do, most breastfeeding mothers find that nursing is a significant aid to weight loss.

Fewer Menstrual Cycles

The hormonal changes that occur with lactation produce a state called *lactation amenorrhea*, which simply means the absence of menstrual periods due to breastfeeding. (See page 84, Chapter 5.) The most prominent advantage of this natural change is its simple convenience. No periods to try to predict, no cramping and a decreased chance of becoming pregnant. (See page 85, Chapter 5 to understand how to employ this in your birth control planning.) And if you are not having periods, you will not be as prone to anemia due to the loss of blood each month.

Also, there may be a correlation between fewer menstrual periods and a lower incidence of cancer of the reproductive system. In cultures where the normal reproductive pattern of a woman is to begin menstruating late, bear a child soon, nurse for an extended period, have a few periods, conceive again, nurse and so on, the incidence of cancer of the reproductive system is very low. Certainly, other cultural factors also contribute to this, but we cannot discount the fact that in our culture, women subject their bodies to more menstrual periods and less breastfeeding. Many researchers believe this to be a prime factor in our society's high rate of cancer of the reproductive system.

Beneficial Hormone Release

The two hormones that are active in lactation, prolactin and oxytocin, offer some advantages to the mother. How these hormones direct the production of milk will be explained in Chapter 3.

Oxytocin. If a mother nurses immediately after birth, the release of oxytocin causes the uterus to contract, helping to expel the placenta. This can take place even if the baby does not catch on to nursing right away and only nuzzles the nipple. Good, strong postpartum contractions are vital to preventing hemorrhage, since they help to close off the capillaries that were left open when the placenta separated. The cramping that accompanies these contractions may be uncomfortable, but the more you nurse, the faster your uterus will return to its pre-pregnancy size. And the faster your uterus shrinks, the faster your abdomen will look fit again.

Oxytocin, which is also the hormone that causes the milk to flow through the duct system, is sometimes called "nature's tranquilizer." Although a new mother (or even an experienced one!) may feel harried and overworked, as soon as she sits down to nurse her baby, her body provides her with a free dose of this wonderful tranquilizer, which probably explains why occasionally mothers might almost drift off to sleep as they nurse their babies in the middle of the day.

Prolactin. Prolactin, the hormone that causes milk to be produced, is also called the mothering hormone, because it contributes to the warm feelings a mother will experience when she sits and caresses her baby. This hormone is so strong, in fact, that when it was given in tests to roosters bred to fight, they could not be induced to do so. It is comforting to know that although you may not feel motherly at first, nature will help you out.

Convenience

Although a bottlefeeding mother often says that she just did not want to go to all the bother of breastfeeding, most breastfeeding mothers cannot quite figure out just what bother she is referring to. Breastfeeding seems the easy winner in terms of convenience. Just pull up your blouse and the meal is ready—sterile, warm and pre-mixed.

• Breast milk is obviously quite portable and is ready any time, any place. No refrigeration or heating is needed.

• Even now when most women just pop bottles into the dishwasher instead of sterilizing them, care of breastfeeding equipment is easier. Most women we know take daily showers!

• Do you ever leave the house, plan to be back in one hour, and find yourself still out four hours later? No problem if you are breastfeeding. But planning for those unforeseen contingencies could be a bother if you have to pack enough extra bottles every time, just in case.

• Night nursings may feel like a real bother to any new parent, since she may have images of the time when most mothers bottlefed and had to get up each time, pad off to the kitchen, prepare a bottle and then go to the baby. However, many nursing mothers find that night nursings become their special quiet time; they simply tuck the baby in bed beside them and nurse and doze away the night, warm and comfortable. (No, you will not roll over onto your baby—more on that later.)

Advantages of the Nursing Relationship

There are incredible rewards to be gained from the relationship that develops between the breastfeeding mother and her baby.

Frequent Contact

One of a baby's most acute senses is her sense of touch. An infant is a very social being, who learns a great deal about her world from frequent, loving contact with those who love her most. Her need for human contact and affection is easily as great as her need for food and care. This frequent contact cements her first loving relationships, which form the basis for life-long emotional health.

• A baby needs to learn to trust that her needs will be met, in order to be able to be trusting as an adult. Frequent contact, combined with the fact that breastfeeding satisfies so many needs, is powerful in developing trust. This early trusting relationship with her mother becomes a cornerstone in her emotional development.

• Breastfeeding ensures that an infant will have lots of contact with her mother and will feel that she is valuable and worthy of love, which she needs to know in order to be able to give love as an adult.

• Frequent loving contact affirms a baby's sense of value, which leads to the development of healthy self-esteem, a crucial factor behind both her emotional well-being and her ability to develop healthy relationships throughout her life.

We cannot say, of course, that bottlefeeding precludes love in any way. A bottlefed baby certainly learns to love her mother, too. But the very nature of breastfeeding makes certain that the contact and attention cannot be denied. It is nature's insurance that this loving relationship will develop.

Bonding

Maternal-infant bonding, the process by which mother and baby form an attachment, has many of the characteristics of falling in love. As a mother and baby bond, they stroke, coo and gaze lovingly into each other's eyes. During a newborn's early stages of quiet alertness, she and her mother have the time to get to know one another leisurely and to fall in love. Bonding can take place without breastfeeding, of course, but breastfeeding can play an important part in this process.

• The first element in the bonding process is eye-to-eye contact. Newborns can see quite well, but their eyes are focused at a range of ten to sixteen inches, just the distance between a mother's face and a baby's when they are nursing. Also, babies naturally seek out a human face to look at, even in the very early days. Studies show that when infants are offered a choice of a random geometric form or the form of a human face, they invariably choose to look at the face.

• Another element that facilitates bonding is skin-to-skin contact. The skin is one of a newborn's most receptive organs, and lots of stimulation through breastfeeding, caressing and stroking is certainly in order. The baby is very receptive to this active demonstration of affection that encourages the love between her and her mother to flourish.

• Some women experience bonding almost like "super-glue." They fall in love with their babies almost immediately and feel incredibly attached to them. Other women, however, may expect too much and find themselves disillusioned when they do not instantly fall in love. Remember that bonding is an attachment *process*, and it can take place instantly or over a period of time.

Mothering Skills

Breastfeeding contributes specifically to a cycle of positive reinforcement. It offers the mother a multipurpose tool with which to meet her baby's needs. As she meets these needs, she

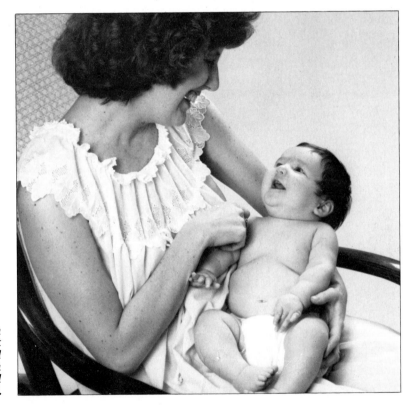

Breastfeeding can play an important part in how you and your baby create a loving and lasting bond.

feels confident as a mother, and the baby feels loved. A lovable baby encourages the mother to continue the love relationship, and the cycle goes on. This cycle may be responsible for the remarkable differences that have been noted between the way breastfeeding and bottlefeeding mothers react to their babies.

• A breastfeeding mother seems to have far less tolerance for the sound of her baby crying. Crying is more disturbing to her, and she responds more quickly to it. This fact sometimes scares a new mother, who envisions her new baby becoming "spoiled" and crying more often because she knows her mother will come running immediately. A study has shown, however, that when a baby is picked up and comforted quickly rather than being allowed to cry, crying becomes less a part of that baby's behavior. She knows she can trust that someone will come and meet her needs quickly, so a great deal of crying is not necessary.

• Other studies show some differences in everyday behavior habits developed by the mothers of breastfed and bottlefed babies. Bottlefeeding mothers are likely to jiggle and pat their babies to comfort them and are more worried about their babies having gas. Breastfeeding mothers, in contrast, tend to make more use of comforting behaviors like stroking and rocking, and they kiss their babies more often.

Chapter Two
Before Your Baby Arrives

A rmed with the desire to breastfeed your baby, and the commitment and motivation that come with the knowledge of its advantages, you have already begun the most important preparation for successful breastfeeding. But there are additional steps you can take before your baby is born to guarantee that you get off to the best possible start. Breastfeeding is natural, but some advance education, communication with involved parties, and physical preparation will ensure that nature has a chance to take its course.

Learn More

Many forms of education are now available to new parents. Evaluate them carefully, keeping your personal desires in mind, and then take advantage of all of the educational opportunities you can afford. You can never know too much.

• La Leche League is the international group devoted to providing information and support to women who want to breastfeed. It is recognized as the world's leading source of up-to-date and accurate information about breastfeeding. League information is primarily down-to-earth and very practical, but it also has access to very technical and scientific information, should you need it. La Leche League group meetings are the best source of information and support available to any new mother.

• More and more specialized classes are becoming available to new parents. In most communities of any size, you can find classes on childbirth, breastfeeding, parenting, adjustment to parenthood, infant massage and many other issues of interest to new parents. Check with area hospitals and clinics, local community schools or universities, and organizations like the YWCA to see what they have to offer.

• We could not begin to name all the books of value. Any reading you do during pregnancy will be of value to you once your baby has arrived. Although many mothers imagine lots of leisure time to read once the baby is home, that is rarely the case.

Communicate With Your Partner

Although good communication is always vital to a relationship, pregnancy is a particularly good time to make sure that you and your partner are really in touch with each other. You were raised in very different households, by very different parents. The only way that you will understand the other's past experience is to talk about it. Discuss at great length the parenting each of you experienced, and the parts you liked and disliked. Take time to sort out your opinions and philosophies about parenting. Each of you will have a set of expectations surrounding the arrival of your new baby; that is natural. But unless you express those expectations clearly to each other, you may be surprised to find that your partner's expectations are different from your own. The following list contains examples of issues you might discuss in order to reveal your preconceptions:

• Will the baby sleep in our bed?

• Who changes a diaper during the night?

• Who does the laundry?

• Who does the grocery shopping?

• Will we both go to doctor appointments?

• Can Aunt Mary babysit, or is she too old?

• Which grandmother will hold him first?

• Shall we take him to bridge club, get a sitter, or quit the club?

• Who will bathe the baby?

• If he is sick, who stays up all night with him?

• Must we budget for all new clothes, or will hand-me-downs do?

• Do we need a baby swing? Can we afford one?

Get the picture? Take time to let your expectations be known; you may be in for a few surprises. Of course, things you have not planned for will continually come up, but the more you know about each other's expectations before the birth, the better off you will be.

Select Your Health-Care Provider

The type of health care you choose and the persons you select to provide it will have a significant impact on your health, happiness and even finances. In order to choose wisely, you need to understand the variety of health care options available and how to choose individuals you'll feel comfortable with.

Types of Health Care Available

Traditional care from an obstetrician (for you) and a pediatrician (for your baby) is still the norm, but many forms of alternative care are becoming more popular and their merits more readily accepted. What some regard as nontraditional care, others find to be excellent, appropriate care for their family and lifestyle. Do not overlook alternative kinds of care as you begin to evaluate health-care providers for your family.

For the Baby. For their new baby's care, many parents prefer a pediatrician, who is trained specifically in the care of children. Another possibility, an M.D. in family practice, appeals to many families today. This doctor, who would treat all members of your family, may be a good choice for a breastfeeding pair because the related needs of mother and baby are handled by the same person. There does seem to be value in being regarded as a family, instead of mother's uterus, baby's colic and father's foot.

For the Mother. While you are breastfeeding, you may need medical attention yourself, for problems ranging from sore nipples or breast infections to back pain. If what you need is breastfeeding information or advice, call your La Leche League Leader or your childbirth educator. If you need treatment, go to your health-care provider, not your baby's. Your health professional might be a gynecologist, a family practice M.D., a chiropractor, a nurse practitioner, a nutritionist or another alternative practitioner.

You will need to spend some time investigating all of the options available. You may decide that just one health-care professional is necessary or that a combination of two or more will satisfy your specific needs the best. No matter what type of care you eventually pick, there are three basic rules that always apply to your relationship with the caregiver.

1. *You* are the consumer. You employ this professional just as you hire a plumber or an accountant.

2. *You* bear the ultimate responsibility for your health. Educate yourself and take an active part in decisions concerning the health of you and your family. Never accept advice from any professional as a divine command. Ask as many questions as it takes to fully answer any concern you have, and feel free to disagree.

3. If, in your relationship with this person, you feel dissatisfied or uncomfortable about the quality of your care, you can always change. Many people feel uncomfortable changing doctors, but would not hesitate finding a new accountant if they were not satisfied with the service of the first one. The same rule applies: if you are not happy, hire someone new.

What to Look for in a Health-Care Provider

It is important that you feel comfortable with your health-care provider's philosophy and personality. Take the time to find someone you respect and trust, and take your "gut-level" reaction into consideration.

You will want a health-care provider who

• recognizes the value of breastfeeding, and considers it before prescribing treatment for a medical problem you might have. He or she should allow you, as a parent, to make choices about breastfeeding, weaning and your style of parenting.

• is personally recommended by a like-minded friend who *uses* this health-care professional.

• respects you, your feelings and your opinions.

• respects the value of your time. If scheduling is done in a way to maximize the doctor's profits but keep you waiting long periods of time, you should feel insulted.

• returns phone calls promptly.

• has good communication skills, and volunteers information and advice so you do not have to pull it out of him or her.

• has partners you find competent and feel comfortable with.

• has a payment policy you can manage. Does the practice demand payment at the time of the visit? Will they bill you? Will they bill your insurance company? (Unfortunately, your insurance coverage may be another factor in your choice. It may not pay for all types of health care.)

• is comfortable when you ignore advice that he or she gives that is not health-related. You should be given credit for being able to make responsible and appropriate parenting decisions. If the advice you receive is on subjects such as weaning, starting solids, comforting vs. ignoring a crying baby, or discipline, you can feel justified in choosing to consider or ignore the advice. *You* are the parenting expert on your child.

How to Interview a Prospective Health-Care Professional

In addition to receiving a personal recommendation and forming your own general impressions, it is very useful to interview a prospective health-care professional. Most good professionals welcome a consultation visit and will be happy to tell you about their practice and philosophy. Here are some practical guidelines to use in preparing for your interview:

• Be confident, not humble. Although you may not know as much about health care as he or she does, you are the consumer; you pay for his or her skills. It is your right and responsibility to select health care that will satisfy your personal goals.

• Make a list of questions before you go. Include issues of philosophy, medical procedures or practice, and even office policy. With a thorough list, you will appear more confident, feel more confident and be less likely to waste any of the professional's time.

• Follow up a question with more questions until you have the information you need. When you ask a question, you will often find that the answer sounds more like reassurance than information. For example, you may ask a prospective pediatrician "Are you in favor of breastfeeding?" Every single pediatrician will say "Yes, I am very much in favor of breastfeeding." In order to discover what you really want to know, follow up with more specific questions. Answers to the following questions might give you a better idea of how this practitioner really manages those mothers who are breastfeeding.

What percentage of mothers in your practice leave the hospital breastfeeding?

What percentage are still breastfeeding at six months? At one year?

What would you advise if I felt my milk supply was low?

How do you treat jaundice in the newborn? (See page 118, Chapter 7, for information on neonatal jaundice.)

Will you write orders for demand feeding and for no supplemental formula or water for my baby while we are in the hospital?

Under what circumstances might you recommend supplementing with or weaning to formula?

If you ask a question about weaning, for instance, beware of answers like "Only if it is absolutely necessary." What does that mean? Who decides when it is absolutely necessary? Can you give me specific examples of what you consider to be absolutely necessary reasons for weaning?

• Observe the health-care provider's reaction to your questions as the interview proceeds. You will be hoping to find someone who is interested in providing accurate responses to your concerns and who is happy that you are informed and eager to participate in your baby's health care. At the same time, beware of the person who is so eager to please that he serves his practice like a famous hamburger—"Have it your way." You may encounter a difficulty that *does* require some active support from your professional, and if he or she has no personal conviction about the merits of breastfeeding, you may not find the encouragement you need to maintain that important breastfeeding relationship. On the other hand, if the care provider seems defensive, insulted or threatened, take this as a clue to this person's personality and style of communication. It may also indicate an insecurity about his or her knowledge and capabilities. You have the information you need; keep looking.

Finding appropriate and capable care can be difficult. The world is full of competent health-care professionals, but since health care is a matter of individual preferences, you may need to arduously investigate all the possibilities. We assure you, the end result of a confident and trusting relationship with a person you respect is well worth the effort.

Perform a Prenatal Breast Self-Exam

Many health-care professionals do not perform prenatal breast exams or at least do not share information with the mother about a breast exam they might perform. Because an exam can be reassuring and can catch potential problems early, we think a self-exam using the following guidelines is a good idea.

Size. Many small-breasted women worry about their ability to produce milk, but breast size is related to the amount of fat in the breast, not to the number of duct systems present. Breast size will not be a factor in your ability to breastfeed. If you have very large breasts, however, you may have to support your breast during feedings in the early months. A small baby will not have the strength to keep a large, heavy breast in place with suction alone. You might also need extra support in a bra during both pregnancy and lactation.

Different-Sized Breasts. Many women have breasts that are not exactly the same size. This is usually not a concern. A dramatic difference in size, however, can sometimes indicate a problem in the development of glandular lobes, which *could* possibly affect your ability to produce milk. This is extremely rare, however.

Nipples. You should be conscious of the protractability of both nipples. Do they protrude or are they flat or almost flat? Are

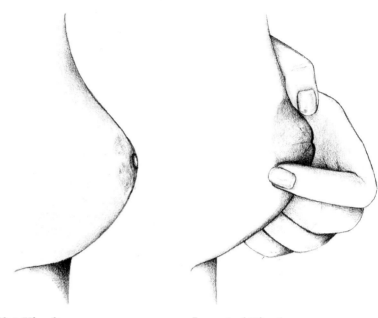

Sometimes these conditions do not cause a nursing problem. If they do, it is easy to manage. (See page 106-108 for management techniques.)

Flat Nipple　　　　**Inverted Nipple**

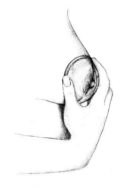

Breast Shield

Exerts an even and continuous pressure which will gradually help to draw out your flat or inverted nipples.

they visibly inverted or do they retract if you squeeze on the area behind the nipple? If so, they are called inverted nipples. If you have flat or inverted nipples, you should wear breast shields during your pregnancy. (Keep in mind that these conditions do not always cause a nursing problem, and even if they do, it is fairly easy to manage.) (See page 107 for illustration and management techniques.)

Unless you are preparing flat or inverted nipples with nipple shields, no other physical preparation for breastfeeding is necessary. Techniques like pulling, rolling or rubbing the nipples will neither help nor harm you. Rubbing your nipples with a towel, however, can actually contribute to soreness by removing the natural oils that nature has provided for your nipples, which results in tough, less elastic nipple tissue that will become sore when stretched into the back of the nursing baby's mouth.

Breast Change During Pregnancy. It is normal for your breasts to become larger and more tender during pregnancy. This change, which is more dramatic in some women than in others, indicates that your glandular tissue is developing and responding to hormonal changes. In addition, your nipples and areola will normally darken during pregnancy, and you may notice drops of colostrum leaking during the last few months. No breast changes at all during pregnancy might indicate a potential problem in your ability to produce milk.

Breast Surgery. Most breast surgeries—including a biopsy, breast enlargement or breast reduction—will not interfere with your ability to nurse. There are two exceptions to this, however: if your nipple was removed and replaced during surgery or if an extensive incision was made along the outside of the areola. A noticeable decrease in nipple sensation after this surgery could mean that essential nerves were cut and your ability to produce milk may be decreased. (For more information about the implications of this, see page 129.)

There is a large range of what is normal for breasts, and the possible deviations we refer to are rare. Most breasts of any shape or size are normal and work well during lactation. In fact, research indicates that 95 percent of all women are capable of breastfeeding.

Prepare Your Household

You may wonder what preparing your house has to do with successful breastfeeding. Lots! Although breastfeeding is simple and natural, it is easier if you get off to a good start. You will be learning to nurse at a time when there is increased stress in your life—the presence of a new baby—so if you and your household are well prepared in advance, the stress can be greatly relieved, and your time and energy can be fully directed toward the beginning of successful breastfeeding.

Arrange for Help
You will need help when your new baby arrives, but that help does not have to be the usual mother or mother-in-law. The idea is to have *household* help, *not* baby help. Your mother or mother-in-law is the best choice only if she will take care of as much of the household work as possible so that you can spend all of your time resting and nursing your baby.

Choose someone who will come in and take over all aspects of running your household. It can be almost as difficult making decisions and preparing grocery lists as it would be to do the actual work and shopping yourself. Let your helper do it all for you, and concentrate on the luxury of having time to spend nursing your baby instead. Be prepared, with someone else running your home, to have things done in a way that may not be your way. Do not worry that the spoons may end up where the knives belong.

Here are some possibilities:

• Some people find that a sister or cousin who has had children is very good help, because she may have breastfed her baby. (Many of our mothers' generation have not.) She may also feel less like an authority figure, so she will allow you more room to make your own decisions about how to care for the baby.

• Many couples find that having the father home for a few weeks is the best choice. Most fathers are quite capable of running a household, and they know where the knives and spoons go. This choice offers the new family time to get started as a family, without outside influence. It also offers the father a wonderful time to get to know his new baby and to participate in the beginnings of the breastfeeding relationship.

• Trade cooking responsibilities with a neighbor or friend. You cook for her family for two weeks of meals any time during your pregnancy, and she in turn feeds your family for the first two weeks after your baby is born. The same plan works well for cleaning.

• Even a young teenager or pre-teen can be a lot of help for little money. He or she can come in every day after school and fold laundry, make a salad for dinner, run errands, or wash dishes and set the table. Teenagers are always eager to be employed; they work for less money than professional help, and they also love to be involved with the advent of a new baby.

• If you have money to spend on professional help, spend it on a cleaning service and ready-made meals, *not* on a nurse for the baby. Think about it for a minute. Would you rather be washing the kitchen floor while some stranger takes your baby out for a walk, or would you rather have someone else be washing that floor while you and your baby curl up together for a nursing and nap?

• If friends throw a shower for you and ask what types of things you need, suggest this idea: each of the women at the shower could donate one or two days of care for your house when the baby comes. You save them the money they would have spent on gifts, each of your special friends gets to spend a day or two in your home with the new baby, and you receive a present that is worth a hundred times the cost of a stretch suit.

No matter what you eventually arrange, remember that your helper's attitude is more important than how they are related to you or how much they are paid. You need someone truly supportive of your breastfeeding, which may mean someone who has done so herself or at least is very enthusiastic about your decision to breastfeed. And you need household help that will help with the household and allow you to mother.

Clean and Organize Your Home

Your natural urge in late pregnancy will probably have you wanting to make your home as clean and appealing a place as possible for the arrival of your baby. As long as you do not tire yourself, take advantage of this natural "nesting instinct."

• If you are so inclined, go ahead and give your home one good cleaning. You may find that your priorities change after the baby is born, and it may be some time before your house sees this kind of cleaning again. Of course, once your baby arrives, your kitchen and laundry must be kept up—you have to eat and have clothes to wear. But the dusting and vacuuming will often go undone. If you anticipate that and realize that other things are simply more important now, it will be easier on your mental health.

• Pay some attention now to preparing for the baby's presence. Plan the baby's room for efficiency, not decor. Make up the crib in layers—mattress pad, rubber pad, sheet, then another rubber pad and sheet, then another pair. If your baby spits up or his diaper leaks, you just gather him in your arms, pull off the soiled pair, and lay him back down on fresh linens. They are even still warm!

• Plan another changing area or two in other parts of the house—going to his room to change him when you are tired feels like a marathon. Keep each area equally well stocked with supplies.

• Keep an additional stock of baby (and mother) things at your bedside too. A few diapers, a pitcher for water, washcloths, a nightgown and many rubber pads kept there will save you countless trips in the middle of the night.

• Arrange a movable bed of some type. A bassinet on wheels, a baby carriage, a car bed or anything else portable will allow your baby to sleep near you, wherever you happen to be in your home.

Breastfeeding itself requires little or no preparation, but time spent now to prepare your household for the arrival of your baby will be very worthwhile. When your baby comes home you will be able to devote all your time and energy to him and to the beginning of successful breastfeeding.

You have educated yourself, chosen health care, and prepared your household for the arrival of your baby. You are truly ready to carry out your decision with the least amount of trouble. Well prepared means well on your way to success!

Chapter Three

The Amazing Breast

T he breast is a fascinating, complex gland that is governed by a system of hormones and physical stimulants to manufacture and secrete nutrition (in the form of milk) to the human infant. Understanding how this system works and the physiology and anatomy of the breast will increase your confidence in your ability to breastfeed.

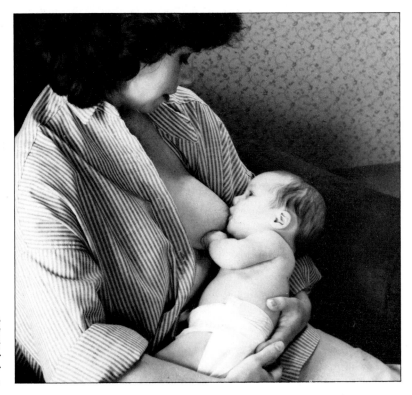

Understanding the physiology and anatomy of the breast will increase your confidence in your ability to breastfeed.

Hormones

The Menstrual Cycle

As a young girl grows up, her breasts and duct system grow. Even before puberty she begins to produce estrogen and progesterone, the two hormones that control her reproductive system. The regular monthly menstrual cycle of a woman is based upon a complex balance of many different hormones, the primary ones being estrogen and progesterone. Each cycle, divided into four phases, is governed by how these hormones act and react to one another.

Phase 1

The bleeding phase is the beginning of a woman's menstrual cycle. During this phase, which usually lasts just under one week, a woman sheds the tissues that have thickened in preparation for receiving a fertilized egg. Estrogen and progesterone remain at low levels.

Phase 2

During the proliferative phase, a slight and gradual rise in the level of progesterone causes the lining of the uterus to grow thicker, or proliferate, in preparation for the presence of an egg. Although the progesterone level rises, estrogen is still the predominant hormone in this phase.

Phase 3

Ovulation, the next phase, occurs about fourteen days before the next period. The estrogen level peaks at this point and then drops abruptly. Most women experience increased sexual drive, and the cervical mucus becomes very wet to facilitate travel of the sperm. This is a woman's most fertile time.

Phase 4

The last phase, the secretory phase, is the most hormonally active of all four phases. After an egg has been released from an ovary, the remnant of the follicle that once contained it (called the corpeus luteum) produces progesterone. This rising level of progesterone causes the lining of the uterus to secrete nourishment for the egg, and the secretory system of the breast begins to prepare for lactation.

If You Do Not Conceive.
The corpus luteum regresses and the progesterone level starts to fall, as does the level of estrogen. The low level of progesterone causes the nourishing lining to begin to break down, and within a week it is discharged during Phase 1 of a new menstrual cycle. Your breasts may feel full and tender for the week before your period, until the secreted fluid is reabsorbed.

If You Do Conceive.
The fertilized egg produces a hormone that keeps the corpus luteum active, so the levels of estrogen and progesterone remain quite high. The production of these hormones continues until the placenta is mature enough to begin producing them itself. The levels remain high throughout pregnancy, and your breasts continue to feel full and tender.

During Pregnancy

Once you conceive and are pregnant, estrogen, progesterone, prolactin, and a number of other hormones develop the breast even further; the duct system proliferates and branches, and the glands that secrete the milk form. By the end of the first trimester, prolactin triggers the production of colostrum.

During the second trimester, a complicated series of hormonal events causes the breast to develop and prepare for lactation. Colostrum begins to be secreted, and later in pregnancy, under the influence of prolactin, the breast begins to produce what will become the constituents of breast milk. Preparation is then complete.

During Lactation

Just as the hormones estrogen and progesterone govern the reproductive cycle, prolactin and oxytocin are most active during lactation. Both are released by the tactile stimulation of the breast in the form of sucking or nuzzling at the breast by the newborn.

Prolactin, whose very name suggests that it supports (pro) breastfeeding (lactation), is the hormone that is most important to breastfeeding. A variety of factors like stress, exercise, sexual intercourse and nipple stimulation will release extra amounts in both lactating and nonlactating women. It travels in the bloodstream, so the extra blood flow that normally occurs in pregnancy and lactation carries increased amounts of it through a pregnant or breastfeeding woman's system.

Lactation begins at birth, when the placenta, which has been producing progesterone and estrogen, is expelled, and the levels of these two hormones drop abruptly. Although estrogen has enhanced the effect of prolactin in *preparing* the breast for lactation, it inhibits prolactin's ability to *initiate* milk secretion, so the disappearance of estrogen and the presence of prolactin trigger the onset of lactation. If any portion of the placenta were to remain in the uterus after birth, the estrogen in it could prevent lactation from beginning.

How the Breast Gives Milk

When the placenta is expelled and lactation is initiated, milk production begins; the first milk usually comes in about two to four days after birth. The components that were manufactured late in pregnancy are there, ready to go into the milk, and they continue to be made as breastfeeding keeps the levels of prolactin high.

Each time your baby nurses, a number of important and interrelated events occur, all of which are vital to the success of breastfeeding. First, the tactile stimulation of the breast causes the pituitary gland to release prolactin, which keeps the process of milk production going. At the same time, oxytocin is released, causing the myoepithelial cells to tighten around each of the alveoli and to squeeze the milk out and into the ducts, through which it travels to the sinuses. If oxytocin were not active, you could have plenty of milk, but your baby would receive only the small amount that trickled down through the ducts and into the pools.

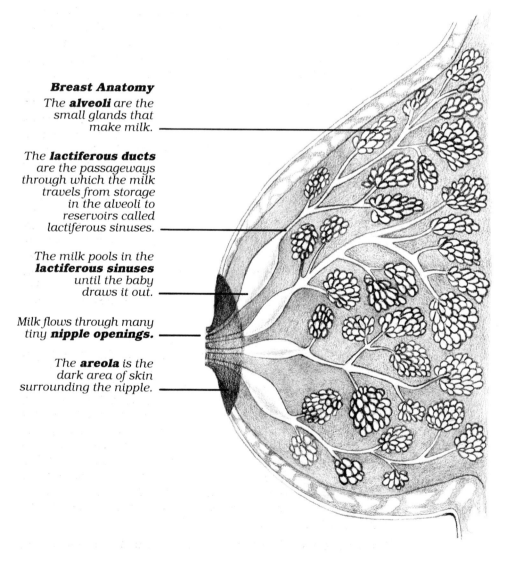

Breast Anatomy

The **alveoli** are the small glands that make milk.

The **lactiferous ducts** are the passageways through which the milk travels from storage in the alveoli to reservoirs called lactiferous sinuses.

The milk pools in the **lactiferous sinuses** until the baby draws it out.

Milk flows through many tiny **nipple openings.**

The **areola** is the dark area of skin surrounding the nipple.

Then, the *pumping* action of the baby's jaws (not the sucking, as most people assume) draws the milk from these sinuses or reservoirs. Your baby must really pull the nipple far back into her mouth so that her gums can compress or squeeze the milk sinuses, literally squirting the milk out and into her mouth. Each time the baby draws the milk out, more flows down.

Let-Down Reflex

The term used to describe the ejection of milk is *let-down*. No matter how much milk your body produces, your baby will not get enough if this reflex does not work properly. It is a basic, crucial element to successful breastfeeding.

Your let-down of milk is usually easily regulated by the act of breastfeeding itself. When the tactile stimulation of the baby at the breast causes the release of oxytocin, you experience the let-down reflex, usually a minute or two after your baby begins to nurse. Let-down of the milk will cause a strong surge of milk, so if the baby is at the breast, she might gulp and swallow quickly for a moment or two, and your breast on the other side may leak. (If your baby is not nursing, both breasts may leak.) The sensation that usually accompanies this surge of milk is often described as a pins-and-needles feeling or a mild tingling in your breast. Other women say that it feels like a very mild ache, or simply a strong sensation of fullness. Almost all women find it a pleasant, not an uncomfortable, sensation, though. It is possible that you may not feel your let-down reflex for the first several weeks. Or you may feel a let-down most of the time for some time; then, several months later you almost never feel it. (This is common as your baby grows older.) The key here is that the *experience* of let-down and the *sensation* of let-down do not always correlate. You may or may not feel it, but it is a rare woman who truly does not have an effective let-down reflex.

In the early weeks, your let-down of milk may not be well coordinated with nursings. You may not experience let-down right after the baby begins to nurse, or you may experience it at odd times between nursings. A sexual climax, for instance, may trigger a let-down. This may evoke some loving chuckles, but it is no real problem and will diminish with time. For many women, the sight, sound or smell of their baby is enough to cause a let-down. You may experience it when you step in to check on your sleeping baby, and you may even have a let-down of milk when you hear a baby cry or you think of your baby. As time passes and your body adjusts to the baby, however, your let-down reflex will become much more regular, occurring only when the baby initiates it.

A few factors can inhibit your let-down reflex from functioning well, or in extreme cases, from working at all. The most common cause is severe psychological or emotional stress. Take life easy, rest and relax as much as possible, and you should have no problem with your let-down reflex. If you are having a let-down difficulty, see page 109 for solutions.

Understanding Milk Supply

Probably the most universal concern among breastfeeding mothers is, "Do I have enough milk for my baby?" When a baby is fed from a bottle, a parent can see just how much the baby drank. Not so with breastfeeding; you have to trust the system and look for more subtle clues to know if your baby is well fed. While many mothers worry about supply, few have any kind of problem with it. Let's see how the system maintains the supply level to understand why this is so.

There is a simple principle behind the fact that mothers can produce the right amount of milk for a very small, weak baby, for a large, hungry baby, or even for twins! Quite simply, the more your baby drinks, the more milk your body will make for her. If she cuts back (she will when she grows older), your body will adjust and cut back as well. It is supply and demand.

Pressure within the breast is your body's clue to the amount of milk your baby takes. When your breast is full and you feel a great deal of pressure, your body knows that the baby has not emptied the breast, so it cuts down on milk production. Conversely, when the breast is soft and your baby has emptied it more completely, this slackening of pressure within the breast cues your body to step up production.

This entire process of receiving the signal to step up production, producing new milk, and having that milk enter the breast takes only 24 to 48 hours to complete. So if by late Wednesday you notice that your baby has been especially hungry that day and your supply seems low, simply nurse her as often as you can, and by Friday morning your supply will catch up to this increased demand. If you ever want to increase your milk supply, put your baby to the breast more often, even if she is not fussing to be fed.

Some women mistakenly try to "save" milk for their baby. If their milk supply seems temporarily low, they may wait longer between nursings, hoping that more milk will accumulate for the next nursing. While this *will* allow the breasts to become full, less milk will be produced. It may seem paradoxical, but mothers who want to *produce* more milk should *nurse* more often and keep their breasts rather empty. Then their bodies will realize that there is not enough milk there and step up production.

Indicators of Low Supply

1. Your baby nurses longer and more frequently than usual.

2. You notice fewer wet diapers a day than normal.

3. Your breasts seem softer, and you leak less than usual.

4. The baby often seems hungry, or appears frustrated at the breast.

Indicators of Plentiful Supply

1. Your baby is happy and healthy.

2. Your baby has six to eight wet diapers a day.

3. Your milk may leak or drip, especially during your let-down reflex.

4. You can hear and see her swallow frequently.

No one of these indicators is foolproof, so never take just one of them as evidence that your supply is low. But most women will notice a pattern or a series of these indications and be able to determine from that if supply is their problem.

Chapter Four Breastfeeding Know-How

We have discussed the benefits of breastfeeding and the mechanics of milk production. Now it is time to explore the practical aspects of making the breastfeeding relationship work. Getting off to a good start with your newborn is an important step that requires developing attitudes conducive to easy and happy breastfeeding. It is also

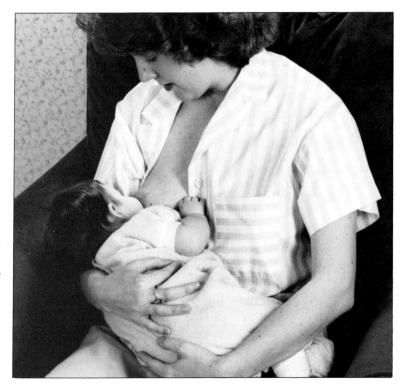

Proper Breastfeeding Position

If you have an idea of what you will receive from (and what you will give to) the breastfeeding relationship, it will become a more comfortable and rewarding experience.

important to understand what the breastfeeding baby is like and what his needs are. If you have an idea of what you will receive from (and what you will need to give to) the breastfeeding relationship, it will become a more comfortable and rewarding experience.

The Basics

Your First Feedings

The very first feeding will probably be in the hospital—in either the labor or recovery room. You may be surprised to discover that your baby is not very interested in nursing at first, but that is fairly common. Many babies are tired. After all, being born is pretty exhausting!

When you attempt this first nursing, you will probably have on a hospital gown, which makes things a little awkward. Remembering to put the gown on backwards before delivery will simplify getting the baby to the breast when the time comes. If you are wearing the gown in the traditional way, you can slip off one shoulder of the gown to facilitate nursing.

One of your birth attendants should help you bring your baby to the breast while you are still on the delivery table; immediate nursing will help expel the placenta and has many other benefits. Nursing right away may be awkward because you will be flat on your back and your baby may nurse only a little. You will be able to settle in for a more comfortable nursing in the recovery room where you can lie on your side.

You may hear from hospital personnel that you do not have any milk in the early days so there is no point in nursing yet. They may offer to feed the baby bottles of formula until your milk comes in.

In reality, however, it is of great value to nurse as soon after birth as possible and nurse frequently in the early days before your milk "comes in."

Your baby may simply "root" (move his head back and forth as he searches for the nipple), and then nuzzle it a little. Even this nuzzling has value, since it will stimulate your milk supply and promote the growth of harmless bacteria on the nipple which protect the infant from harmful bacteria.

If your baby tends to be sleepy, do not worry. Just keep offering your breast and soon he will reward you with a vigorous nursing. Some babies do not seem interested in nursing until 40-72 hours after birth. If a baby does not nurse within the first half hour of life, his sucking urge will probably drop, but will reappear two or three days later.

On the other hand, many babies latch on and nurse eagerly at their first opportunity. They nurse the way you imagined they would, as if they have been taking an intrauterine correspondence course on breastfeeding.

Why Nurse Right Away?

Immediate nursing offers you and your newborn many benefits:

• It provides colostrum, your "early milk," which contains valuable properties, including antibodies, that help protect your infant.

• It aids in establishing the bonding, or emotional tie, between mother and baby.

• It causes uterine contractions, which help to prevent hemorrhaging in the mother and help her uterus begin to return to its pre-pregnancy size.

• It is associated with longer and more successful breastfeeding.

• It aids in establishing the mother's let-down reflex.

• It helps to make the milk ducts more elastic, which may be a factor in preventing breast engorgement.

• It provides your baby with the opportunity to practice breastfeeding on the smaller quantities of colostrum. When your milk comes in, he will be experienced and ready!

Although these early nursings are valuable, do not worry if your baby is not willing to nurse much during the first few days of his life. Babies are born with nutrient and fluid stores that will last until the milk comes in. Once he begins to nurse, he will surely make up for lost time.

Some Hospital Policies

As parents have become more informed about early infant needs and optimal practices that aid bonding and establish successful breastfeeding, they have started to question many hospital practices. Hospitals have been responsive to this pressure and have begun to change some of their maternity policies. Here are some of the practices and issues you should be aware of.

Eye Medication

Most states require hospitals to administer ointment to all infants as a safeguard against eye damage from gonococcal conjunctivitis, a complication that would occur if the mother had gonorrhea. Silver nitrate has been used in the past, but has been replaced with Erythromycin.

One of the side effects of Erythromycin, however, is to temporarily blur an infant's vision. Since eye-to-eye contact is an important element of the bonding process (see page 17), blurring his vision at that time is unwise. Knowing this, you can request that the ointment be delayed until you have had some time, maybe an hour, with your baby. This way the law is observed, but bonding is not disrupted.

Nipple Shields

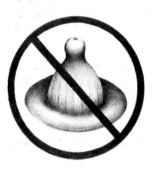

Nipple Shield

They can be detrimental to your nursing efforts. Your baby needs to learn to draw your nipple into the back of his mouth, rather than having a rubber nipple placed there. And, nipple shields may cause your nipples to become sore.

If your baby is a little slow or reluctant at first to latch onto your breast, a well-meaning nurse may offer you a nipple shield, a rubber nipple that's placed over your nipple. Your baby is supposed to latch onto the rubber nipple covering your nipple and to nurse through the shield.

A reluctant baby may latch onto a nipple shield more readily than your nipple because it can be forced into the back of his mouth where his sucking reflex is triggered. But nipple shields are not recommended because they can be extremely detrimental to your nursing efforts. For one thing, your baby needs to learn the knack of *drawing* your nipple into the back of his mouth himself, not having a rubber nipple inserted there. Usually all he needs is time and your patience. Just keep offering, coaxing and trying again. Also, letting your baby nurse on a nipple shield may put pressure on your nipples and cause soreness, since he may be pressing down on your nipple itself, instead of the areola, where milk pumping really should take place.

While there is little value in using a nipple shield, if a nurse insists that you try it, and you are really worried about your baby's slow start, use it only for the minute it takes him to latch on. Then, once he is sucking in rhythm, slip the shield away, and he will usually latch right back onto your nipple without even noticing. Never leave the shield in place for the whole feeding.

Supplementation

It is standard procedure in some hospitals to supplement breastfed babies with either glucose water or formula or both. There are several disadvantages to doing this.

• Most importantly, supplements keep your baby from the breast right at a time when he needs to learn to breastfeed and your milk supply needs to be stimulated.

• Since breast milk and colostrum are the perfect foods for a baby, no formula can duplicate them. Colostrum requires virtually no digestion, so why replace it with an inferior food which will stress your baby's immature digestive system?

• A rubber nipple and a flesh nipple feel very different in the baby's mouth and require two totally different sucking actions. Some babies become confused if faced with both nipples too early. If a baby learns to suck on a bottle early, he may have trouble breastfeeding, but if he masters breastfeeding first, he is likely to adapt to a bottle as well. The safest approach is to avoid rubber nipples for at least six weeks. If, after that time, there is some reason why your baby must take a bottle, there will be less risk of nipple confusion.

• If you have any history of an allergy to cow's milk on either side of your family, be adamant about restricting any supplements, since by delaying your baby's first exposure to cow's milk (in formula) until he is at least a year old, you can probably avoid this very difficult allergy.

• Glucose water has no value for a normal, healthy full-term baby. It interferes with the immunological protection of breast milk, and fills your baby up so he will not want to nurse. A compromise sometimes offered by the hospital staff is sterile water. They may warn you about the possibility of your baby dehydrating. But babies are born with a fluid supply that lasts until your milk comes in.

Since the hospital staff may give your baby supplements without consulting you, have your pediatrician write orders on your baby's chart for no formula and no water. In addition, remind every nurse caring for you or your baby about these orders.

Separation

The most difficult problem that parents face stemming from hospital policy is separation from their baby. Often a newborn is whisked away right after birth for weighing, measuring, cleaning, foot printing, examining and so on. Although you may not be in a position to accompany your baby during these procedures, it is an excellent idea for your partner to follow and stay with the baby at this time. Then the baby is generally brought to you in the recovery room where you will have some peaceful time together. After that, where your baby spends most of his time will have important consequences for breastfeeding.

Nursery. Your baby might be taken to the infant nursery to spend most of his time there during his hospital days. If he is a "nursing baby" he will be brought to you when the nurses think it is time to feed him, and taken from you at a specified time. It will not really feel like he is "all yours" until you get him home. Hospital policies vary about requiring the baby to be cared for in the nursery. If your baby is required to stay in there, do all you can to have the baby brought to you frequently (every two or three hours) and ask to keep him longer than the usual time allotted.

Rooming-in. If you would like to control your feeding and the contact you have with your baby, we strongly suggest "rooming-in," the practice of keeping the newborn baby in the same room with his mother and letting her assume primary responsibility for his care. We cannot over-emphasize the value of this during your hospital stay. Most hospitals offer this as an option.

The first and most important advantage to rooming-in is the assurance that your baby can be fed on demand. Some hospitals still schedule or limit feedings for the babies in the nursery, but if your baby is with you, he can be protected from this scheduling. The other distinct advantage is that you gain confidence and competence as you learn from the nursing staff how to care for your baby. Tasks such as diapering a newborn and caring for the umbilical cord may seem a little difficult and awkward in the beginning. A chance to practice with guidance is most welcome.

Demand Feeding

Demand feeding—feeding the baby whenever he cries—fits well with nature's supply and demand system of milk production. Since your baby can regulate the amount of nourishment he receives by the frequency and length of his nursings, he can always be assured of having the right amount of milk to meet his nutritional needs. And since he can control the nurturing time he has, he will also be emotionally well fed. Here are some other facts you should know.

• A new baby needs to be fed at least every three hours. Even if he does not cry, you should offer him the breast. He may be too weak or tired to demand to nurse often enough in the beginning, but you can increase his strength by feeding him more often. Soon he will be able to accurately indicate his hunger.

• A new baby may not be strong enough to take in an adequate amount of milk in a single feeding. He may need many short efforts at nursing in order to draw enough milk out. If he fusses even an hour after his last feeding, he is probably hungry again.

• You may have heard that as you begin to breastfeed you should limit the time you nurse in order to prevent sore nipples. But sore nipples are caused by poor positioning at the breast, not by the amount of time you nurse. Nurse according to your baby's needs, not a stopwatch.

• If your baby is allowed to suck freely, he will be happy and you will have a plentiful supply of milk. In addition, the act of sucking will increase blood circulation to the baby's face and head, contributing to the development of the brain.

Positioning Your Baby at the Breast

Your motivation probably makes the most significant contribution to successful breastfeeding. In practical terms, however, positioning the baby correctly at the breast is the most important factor to the physical success of breastfeeding. Positioning the baby's mouth properly on the breast makes it possible for your baby to get a sufficient supply of milk, and it prevents you from getting sore nipples.

Many new mothers have never actually seen a baby nursing at the breast before their own first child is born, so it is no wonder that first attempts at positioning the baby for a feeding may not go well. Although breastfeeding is natural, the technique needs to be learned.

You can position your baby properly at the breast by following the step-by-step method we present. It may feel orchestrated to follow directions for something as natural as putting your baby to the breast, but after just a few feedings, it will become so automatic you will not even think about it. You want to make sure your nursing habits are good ones.

Most of the time, your baby will let go of the nipple himself when he is finished nursing, but if you want to take him off before he lets go (to change sides, for example), simply slide your finger between your breast and the baby's mouth to break the suction; the nipple will slip easily out of his mouth.

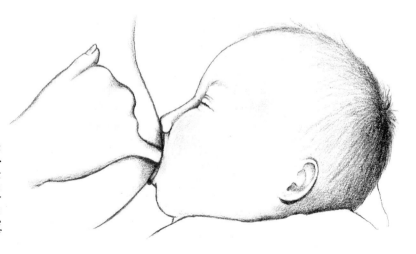

Breaking Suction

Slide your finger between your breast and the baby's mouth to break suction by pressing lightly on your breast. The nipple will slip easily out of his mouth.

Proper Positioning at the Breast

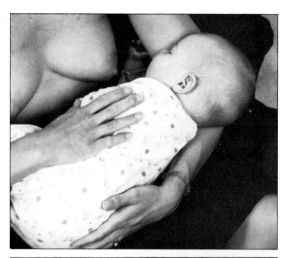

1. Sit down with your baby in a comfortable chair. Place the side of your baby's head in the crook of your arm. Bring the hand of that arm around him. You and your baby should be abdomen to abdomen. Wrap his bottom arm around your side, so it does not get between the two of you.

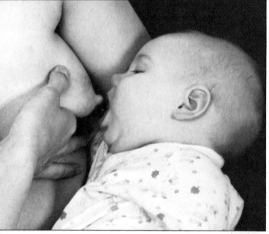

2. Support your breast with your free hand by placing the fingers under your breast and your thumb on top. Keep them all behind the areola.

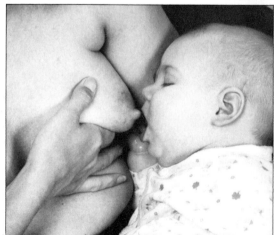

3. Pull your baby close to you. Tickle his upper lip very lightly with your nipple until he opens his mouth wide.

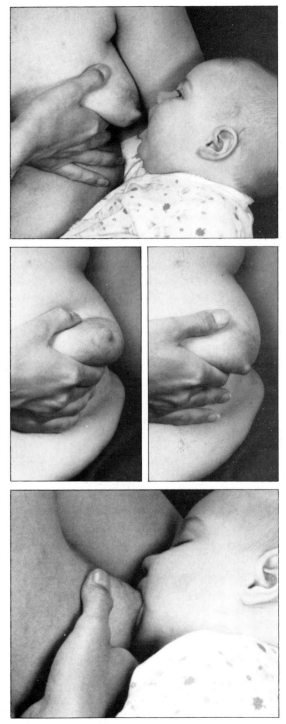

4. Center your nipple and your baby will latch onto it.

5. When centering your nipple, you will be able to alter the position of your nipple by pressing your thumb in to move your nipple up or pressing your fingers in to move it down.

6. When your baby's mouth is on the breast properly, his bottom lip will curl out.

Nursing Postures

Once you have learned the technique for getting your baby onto the breast, you can experiment with various nursing positions other than sitting. The process for helping the baby latch onto the breast is the same regardless of the position.

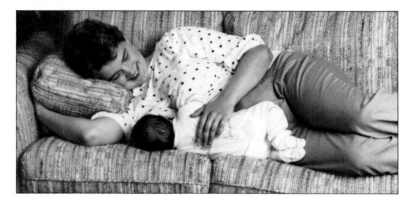

Lying Down

Curl your bottom arm under your head and pull your baby close with your top arm.

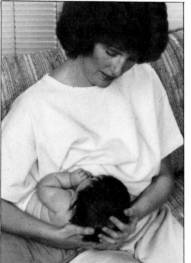

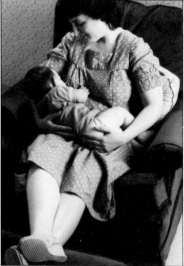

Football Hold

Tuck your baby's legs under your arm toward your back. Hold the back of his head in the palm of your hand. Bring him forward with his face toward your breast.

Back Support

Put your feet up, and position pillows behind you, under your baby or under your arm to bring him up to your breast.

Lying down. Many women find that lying down to nurse is their favorite position, since it is restful and even allows them to nap while their babies nurse. The most comfortable position involves curling your bottom arm under your head and pulling your baby close with your top arm.

The football hold. The "football hold," another nursing posture, can help correct certain difficulties. It can be used, for example, to empty a breast with a plugged duct more efficiently, to relieve some pressure on sore nipples, or to fool a baby who rejects one breast. (See Chapter 7.) Tuck your baby's legs under your arm toward your back. Hold the back of his head in the palm of your hand and bring him forward, with his face toward your breast. If your baby arches in response to feeling your hand against the back of his head, use a blanket between your hand and his head.

The general rule to remember, regardless of what position you use, is this: do not use your muscles for support during a feeding; provide support for yourself so you can relax. Do not lean forward as if to bring the breast to the baby; lean into the back of the chair to help support your back. Put your feet up to make yourself more comfortable. If necessary, use pillows behind you, under your arm, or under your baby to bring him up to your breast.

Burping

It is a good idea to burp your baby after feedings, at least during the first few weeks of nursing. Breastfed babies burp less often than bottlefed babies, since a baby's mouth fits so well around the breast, and air intake is usually not a significant problem. But some do gulp air and definitely need to be burped, while others just will not produce any air in spite of your greatest efforts. After your baby's umbilical cord has fallen off, he can sleep lying on his stomach. At this point burping is not as crucial, because if you lay your full, sleeping baby down on his stomach, any air in there will probably come up by itself.

Since breastfed babies typically fall asleep toward the end of a feeding, we recommend burping your baby as you switch him from one breast to the other. (It is not necessary to wake a sleeping baby for a burp!) Burping between sides has other advantages as well. Your first goal is to bring up air to avoid later digestive discomfort for the baby, but switching sides may stimulate your baby and cause him to become more alert. This alertness may contribute to a more energetic nursing on the second side.

To Burp Your Baby

1. Either lean him over your shoulder, lay him on his stomach across your lap, or sit him up and lean him forward against your hand. Remember to put a diaper under the baby's face, since he may spit up.

2. Then rub or pat his back gently in an upward motion. Even if he spits up quite a bit, do not worry; it is not as much of the feeding as you might think.

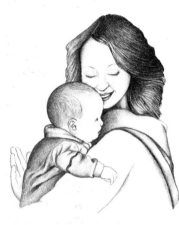 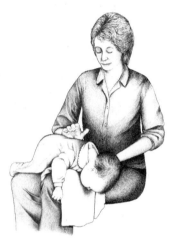 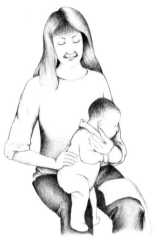

Burping At Shoulder   **Burping Over Knee**   **Burping Sitting Up**

Nipple Care

In addition to good nursing techniques, some added precautions during the early weeks will help prevent sore nipples. If you follow these simple principles, you will probably never have any difficulties. If you do notice any discomfort, however, refer to our section on sore nipples in Chapter 7.

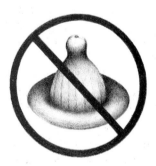

Nipple Shield

Nipple shields often irritate nipples and can interfere with your baby learning to suck properly. Nipple shields should only be used briefly to help the baby grab the nipple.

• To keep your nipples clean, just rinse them with water as you shower or bathe. Never wash them with soap or alcohol or use creams or ointments that contain alcohol, all of which are unnecessary and can dry your nipples.

• During the early weeks, allow your nipples to air dry after each feeding. Leave any breast milk that is still on your nipples and let it dry, since it is good for your skin. Make sure your nipples are dry before pulling up the flaps on your nursing bra.

• Always replace wet or even damp nursing pads, since a moist environment will contribute to sore nipples.

Bowel Movements

Do not be surprised by your breastfed baby's stools. They are usually bright yellow, but can range in color to muddy green, and they can contain some soft curds. As one mother accurately and vividly described them, "They look like mustard and cottage cheese!"

The stools of your breastfed baby may be so soft that you think he has diarrhea. Remember that since a normal stool is very, very soft, his diarrhea would be *extremely* liquid. As long as the color and odor seem right, even a very loose stool can be normal.

During the first two weeks of life, a normal breastfed baby will stool frequently. After that, the frequency of stools will differ from one baby to the next. Some babies move their bowels after every feeding, while others go a very long time between stools—as long as a week. Either extreme can be normal for a totally breastfed baby.

The Nursing Baby

Whenever we see a baby nursing, we always think what a lucky baby he is. When he was born, he found what he was looking for as he "rooted" for the warmth, milk and love that came from his mother's breast. He does what his instincts lead him to do, and he is rewarded with nourishment, health and sensitivity from his mother. We usually see a satisfied, happy baby, who is eager and ready to meet the world.

Nursing Personalities The most important idea we can communicate to you about your baby's personality is that, like all other babies, he is unique. Your baby's individuality is never more in evidence than when he is nursing. Each baby has his very own nursing style—you do not determine or mold it.

Although your baby's nursing personality is his own, we find that babies tend to fall into one of the "categories" we describe below. You may recognize your baby in one or more of these groups. Each one is as normal as the next.

The Go-Getter. This baby is the enthusiastic nurser. He may make overly eager little sounds as the breast approaches. He latches on with strength and nurses with vigor, and he may gulp some air in his attempt to keep up with the let-down reflex. This baby has a strong sucking urge and loves to nurse. You can be sure that when he finishes nursing, he is full.

The Slow Starter. This baby usually causes his mother much anxiety by appearing indifferent to nursing for the first few days after birth. When, much to his mother's relief, he does decide to nurse, he quickly becomes an expert.

The Listless Nurser. This baby may need a little coaxing to latch on. Once he is on, he nurses with little strength and sucks infrequently. He may take long breaks between several weak sucking bouts. This baby will not get his full feeding in twenty minutes; it may even take him an hour to get enough milk to feel full. He may also ask to nurse after only a short interval. Switching sides several times during the feeding will help. (See more on this condition in Chapter 7, page 114.) This baby will become a stronger nurser as he grows.

The Efficient Feeder. This baby settles down to business at the breast. He usually latches on, nurses well for about ten minutes on each side, and then may go as long as four hours between feedings. He does not have a very strong sucking urge.

The Dozer. Only very young infants will display these characteristics. This baby continually dozes at the breast and is very difficult to wake. He may take many incomplete feedings instead of one good one. (See more on this type in Chapter 7, page 115.)

The Snacker. Some babies adopt this style early and may never deviate from it. This baby prefers lots of little nursings to one long, efficient one. Some mothers find this annoying, others enjoy the frequent contact and the playfulness that often accompany these little sessions.

The Clock-Watcher. This baby is not really a very typical breastfed baby. He puts himself on a regular schedule and then may nurse at precise intervals.

The Free Spirit. There is some of this personality in most breastfed babies. Most babies have irregular intervals between feedings, and the length of the nursing probably varies by as much as ten times. One nursing may be a serious quest for food, another a need for comfort or sleep, and another a playful session. On the surface, there may seem to be no rhyme or reason to this baby's nursing pattern, but in reality there is a natural rhythm behind it, and it satisfies his varied needs.

Your baby's nursing style may be your first clue to his gradually unfolding personality, and while you may come to accept your baby's nursing style as the norm, if you have a second child, you will no doubt be introduced to a totally different style.

Nighttime Nursings

Most breastfeeding mothers feel comfortable and confident about meeting their babies' daytime needs. However, nighttime nursings are usually met with more ambivalence and confusion. What about your baby's nighttime needs? Are they less

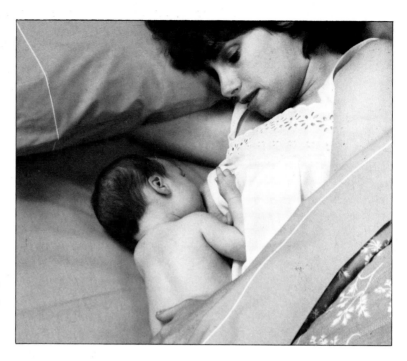

Breastfeeding In Bed

Breastfeeding your baby in bed reassures him that you will meet his needs day or night.

legitimate than those he experiences during the day?

Hardly. It is really the exception more than the rule for a healthy baby to agree to a long period (like eight hours) of solitude and the absence of human contact. It is natural, healthy, and most of all normal, for your baby to need and ask for some human closeness during the night. Whether or not he is actually hungry or thirsty is not the point. Babies need touch and closeness and warmth around the clock. If your baby cries for you during the night, take it as reassurance that your baby has healthy emotional needs and has learned to trust you enough to ask you to meet them.

The easiest way to deal with night wakings is to expect them to be the norm rather than to live for the day your baby will sleep through the night. You will adjust to "punctuated sleep" (sleeping in several short stretches rather than one long one) sooner than your baby will sleep through the night. Make this adjustment your goal.

The Family Bed

Many parents solve the problem of "getting up with the baby" by bringing the baby into bed with them when he first wakes and leaving him in their bed for the rest of the night. Many breastfeeding mothers learn to sleep right through night nursings. Often babies who sleep with their parents wake less because they are warm and secure. Another benefit to keeping the baby in your bed is extra contact time with the father. Bonding and developing a close relationship between baby and father is essential to the happiness of both, and one building block of any relationship is time. Even though both may be asleep, they are aware of each other's breathing, scent and presence. Many fathers love this special time with their babies.

Some Concerns

• **Will you roll over on your baby?** We have never heard of a parent who did. The same instinct that keeps you from rolling off the bed will keep you from rolling onto your baby. Even if you could theoretically roll onto your baby, be assured that he would not lie there passively. He would squirm, cry and wake you.

• **How will having the baby in bed with us affect our sex life?** We suggest bringing your baby in from his bed the first time he wakes; do not start out the night with him in your bed. This gives you and your partner a few hours in bed together before your "family togetherness" time begins.

• **Will my child still be sleeping with us when he is in high school?** The method we suggest, bringing the baby in when he wakes for the first night feeding, will mean that when the baby no longer wakes during the night, he will stay in his own bed all night. If you become uncomfortable having him in your bed before he outgrows the need, compromise a little. Try going to the baby and patting or rubbing his back until he goes back to sleep. Or put his crib mattress on the floor and lay a twin mattress next to it for yourself; when he wakes, you can go to him, lie down next to him, nurse him back to sleep, and then slip back to your own bed.

• **Should we let our baby "cry it out" so that he will "give in" and sleep through the night?** It is true that if you let him cry he *will* eventually "give up" and sleep through the night. But when your baby wakes in the dark with a strong need for his mother, cries for her, and she does not come, he feels terrified, confused and abandoned. The only conclusion his immature mind can draw is that he needs you and you are not there, which is especially upsetting if you have been responsive during the day. A baby needs to know that your love is available to him, regardless of the time of day.

Although on some nights, meeting your baby's needs may feel like a "superhuman" effort, most of the time your family will love this close and cuddly time together. If you feel you need more information and reassurance on the subject of bringing your baby into bed with you, read *The Family Bed*, by Tine Thevinin.

Growth Spurts

All babies experience growth spurts, during which a baby has an instinct and mechanism for increasing your milk supply to meet his growing needs. It is important to understand this mechanism, for although growth spurts are both normal and universal, they are the unfortunate cause of many weanings.

During a growth spurt, your baby will nurse almost continuously for a few days. To meet this additional demand, your milk production system gradually increases the amount of milk available for each feeding. He will then settle comfortably back into his old nursing pattern.

Very often, however, a mother panics at a growth spurt, concludes that she does not have enough milk, and begins supplementing with formula. In reality, she may not have enough milk for him at the start, but if she goes along with her baby's needs and lets him build up her supply the natural way, there would soon be plenty of milk for this growing baby. On the other hand, if she gives formula instead of the extra nursing, her supply will not rise to meet the demand, and she may become dependent on supplements; the bottle may gradually become more the norm than the exception.

Typical times to expect babies to experience growth spurts are

• shortly after your baby comes home from the hospital

• about 6 weeks

• about 3 months

• about 6 months

Keep in mind that these ages are only averages; they are not carved in stone. Your baby has his own growth rate and may experience a spurt at any time. If he increases the frequency or duration of his feedings, follow his lead; he knows what he is doing. He will make sure that you produce precisely the amount of milk he needs if you let him.

Crying

Crying is your baby's most important way of communicating with you. It is meant to disturb you, and your intolerance of it is nature's way of ensuring your baby's survival. You will find that your own baby's cry speaks directly to you—it does not sound like the cry of any other baby. Studies have demonstrated that even a few days after birth, a mother can pick her baby's cry out from the cries of other newborns in the nursery.

Why do babies cry? There are many reasons, but if your baby is breastfed, the first thing most people will say is, "Are you sure the baby is getting enough milk?" A breastfeeding mother's milk supply is always under public scrutiny. However, it would be very unusual for a breastfed baby not to get enough milk. Most breastfeeding mothers have plenty of milk, and most breastfed babies regulate their milk intake to their own satisfaction.

Some of the more probable reasons for an infant crying include the following:

• Discomfort from a wet or soiled diaper, or from being too cold or, more often, too warm.

• An illness like an ear infection, a cold, a stomach disturbance or colic.

• Faulty breathing ability. (Crying can be an emergency breathing technique and calming him will help him to regain control of his immature and faulty breathing ability.)

• Tiredness.

• The need to satisfy his sucking urge. (Some studies have indicated that an infant's desire to suck is even greater than the desire for food.)

• Overstimulation.

• Boredom. Everyone, regardless of age, is miserable when bored.

• The baby's strong need for human contact and attention.

There may be other reasons for crying, but these seem to be the most common. When your baby cries, you may not be able to pinpoint the cause, but it is interesting to point out that to comfort or help your baby with any of these problems, you can offer the same remedy—nursing. Nursing is more than a way of feeding a baby. The breast is meant to be a pacifier as well, and the act of nursing will calm most babies. It is the most wonderful mothering tool available to you.

When You Are Away From Your Baby

It is a fact of modern life that even if you are a breastfeeding mother, you may either occasionally, or regularly if you are employed, need to be separated from your nursing baby. How can you manage this? There are several options to consider.

Leaving a Bottle of Breast Milk

If you need to be away from your baby, you obviously need to leave some milk behind with the caretaker. If you feel it is important to keep your baby on a diet of breast milk exclusively, you can hand-express or pump your breast milk and leave it in a bottle for the baby. If you need to pump milk only occasionally, you have two good choices.

Hand Expression. In order to do this, you need to remember a few guidelines.

• Do not grab your whole breast with your hand and squeeze. This type of pressure can lead to a plugged duct or a breast infection.

• Place your thumb on the top of the areola and your index or your middle finger on the underside. Both fingers should be about one-and-a-half inches behind your nipple. Press your fingers together a few times, then rotate your hand, express again, rotate again, and repeat until you have gone all the way around. These rotations are necessary in order to pump all the lactiferous sinuses.

• Express your milk into a large glass measuring cup. If you lean over to express into it, gravity will assist you. Also, switch sides frequently.

• After pumping, pour the milk into a clean bottle and refrigerate it immediately.

Breast Pump. The second choice is to purchase a small hand pump. We recommend any of the cylinder-type pumps on the market. (See page 79 in Chapter 5 for more on breast pumps.)

Pump after you nurse, so you know your baby has had enough milk first. You will probably need to express several times in order to collect enough milk for a bottle.

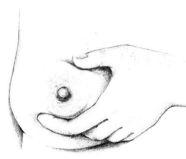 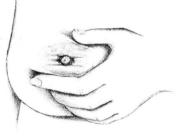

Hand Expression of Milk | *Place your thumb on the top of the areola and your index or middle finger on the underside. Both fingers should be about one-and-one-half inches behind your nipple.* | *Press your fingers together a few times, then rotate your hand, express again, rotate again, and repeat until you have gone all the way around.*

Storing Breast Milk

Breast milk can be stored in either the refrigerator or the freezer. Always label your stored milk with the date of the oldest pumping. In order to store breast milk safely, observe these guidelines about how long you can store it.

Where	*How Long*
In the refrigerator	Two days
In the freezer compartment of a refrigerator	Two weeks
In a freezer that goes below zero degrees	Two years

If you are adding new breast milk to a bottle of frozen milk, cool it in the refrigerator for thirty minutes first. Warm milk would thaw the top layer of what is frozen and, once thawed, breast milk should not be refrozen.

To thaw breast milk, hold the bottle under running tap water that is first cool, then tepid, then warm. When the breast milk is completely liquid, it can be heated either in a pan of water on the stove or under hot tap water. Never let breast milk thaw at room temperature. Once it is thawed, breast milk is good, refrigerated, for four hours. For more information on this subject, read our book *The Breastfeeding Guide for the Working Woman.*

Leaving a Bottle of Formula

If you do not want to express breast milk, you can leave a bottle of formula when you go out. If you are supplementing regularly, as in the case of an employed mother, we would recommend that you try cow's-milk-based formulas first, since they are more nutritious than the soy formulas. If you suspect that your baby might have an allergy to cow's milk, you can try a soy formula.

On the other hand, if you use only an occasional bottle, the formula plays a very small role in your baby's overall nutrition. You could then leave a soy formula in order to avoid early exposure to cow's milk. Be aware, however, that some babies are also allergic to soy.

If your baby objects to taking the bottle from the caregiver, suggest that she give the milk from a syringe, an eye-dropper or a spoon instead.

Principles for Successful Breastfeeding

Throughout our many years of contact with breastfeeding women, we have come to realize that a certain set of attitudes characterizes the successful nursers. These attitudes, in addition to the support and validation that breastfeeding friends can provide, are conducive to a more relaxed and positive approach to breastfeeding.

1. Be Committed and Motivated

Women who understand the benefits of breastfeeding and have a strong desire to succeed are almost always successful. In our experiences we have seen unmotivated women wean their babies for trivial reasons, and we have also seen highly motivated women persevere through difficulties no ten women should have faced. Women often feel a greater sense of motivation and commitment if others reinforce and encourage their desire to breastfeed.

2. Throw Away the Clock

Mothers whose breastfeeding experience is pleasant and easy have a total disregard for the clock. When asked, "How many times a day does your baby nurse?" most experienced breastfeeding mothers know the only possible answer is, "I don't have any idea."

3. Meet Your Baby's Needs

Secure parents with some understanding of their baby's needs are eager to meet them. If you realize that a baby's desires and needs are one and the same, you will feel comfortable with this attitude. Babies do not have the sophisticated mental skills that some parents ascribe to them: there is no reason to be afraid that your baby might want to control or manipulate you. Your baby is a small bundle of needs, and he depends on you to meet them.

Many new parents worry that if they go to their baby every time he cries to be held, they will "spoil" him. You cannot spoil your baby by loving him and satisfying his needs. A wise pediatrician we know gives the following advice to the parents in her practice, "Life un-spoils us so much . . . . so go ahead and hold and love and spoil your baby now."

If an infant's need for closeness is denied, he will never be free of that need, just as if you deny yourself food, your hunger will become so great it will interfere with every aspect of your life. But if his needs are fulfilled, he will be free of them and can go on to be a secure and productive person. Do not be afraid to satisfy your baby's needs. He does not want to control you, he just wants to grow. See his emotional and developmental needs as important, and feel confident in your ability and responsibility to satisfy them.

4. Let Your Milk Supply Become Established

One trait successful breastfeeding mothers share is a worry-free milk supply, something they gave themselves time to really establish in the beginning. You can assure yourself of a good supply if you have a clear understanding of the supply-

and-demand system of milk production, and, if at all possible, you hold off on any pumping or supplementing for six weeks after the birth of your baby.

5. Be Comfortable Nursing Away from Home

Comfort with the idea of nursing away from home is necessary to the on-the-go lifestyle of many breastfeeding mothers. One convenience of breastfeeding is that your baby's food is always with you, but as a new mother nursing away from home, you may be self-conscious. You need to realize that you can nurse without exposing your breast. Nurse by pulling your blouse up from the bottom, not unbuttoning from the top.

Practice nursing in front of a mirror at home, to reassure yourself that you are not exposed. Then, with experience, you will gradually become comfortable nursing in public, whether in restaurants, movie theaters, airplanes, stores, parks or just about anyplace! And because you can learn to nurse discreetly, do not worry about offending anyone by nursing in public. Although many people are uncomfortable seeing an exposed breast, no one should object to the idea that the baby is being

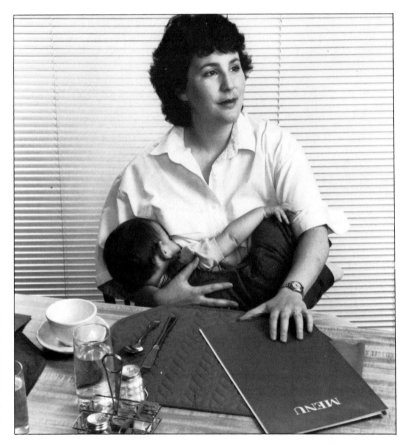

Discreet Nursing

You can nurse without exposing your breast. Pull your blouse up from the bottom. Do not unbutton from the top. With experience, you will gradually become comfortable nursing in public.

fed if they cannot see the breast. In fact, by nursing discreetly in public, you are actually helping society get used to the idea that breastfeeding is normal and natural, and you are doing it in a way that is easy to accept.

This expertise in nursing away from home contributes to successful nursing in two ways. First, you are happy with the ease of breastfeeding rather than resentful of any restrictions. Secondly, you are not interfering with your milk supply by leaving the baby home with a bottle, bringing a bottle along, or making your baby wait to nurse after he is hungry. Instead, you can continue to happily nurse on demand wherever you go. A breastfed baby rarely causes a public disturbance, regardless of where you take him—he can always be comforted and quieted within seconds.

The Breastfeeding Mother

Chapter Five

When you begin to nurse, you enter one of the most rewarding and enjoyable times of your life, a period often characterized by an intense level of caregiving. Most women receive great satisfaction from this unique opportunity to give and be the center of their baby's universe.

It is also typical, however, to focus so entirely on the baby that you tend to put your own needs aside altogether. But if you go into this period understanding what your needs will be and take care to meet them, you will enjoy breastfeeding more. Use the information in this chapter to meet your practical, physical and emotional needs.

Diet

Lactation does not place a great strain on a woman's body and it does not generate huge dietary needs. There is, however, a great deal of confusion about the subject of the breastfeeding woman's diet. How much should you eat? Can you diet? What foods are essential for producing milk? Which foods should you avoid? We hope to clarify and simplify these and other diet-related issues.

Caloric Needs

Your body needs to expend approximately 600 to 800 calories a day for the components of breast milk and the energy it takes to produce them. The fat you stored during pregnancy should supply about 300 calories a day. Therefore you need to eat enough additional food to supply the remaining 300 to 500 calories per day. But you probably will not need to make an effort to add these extra calories to your diet; you will find that you are naturally hungrier.

Your body produces milk quite efficiently. About 90 percent of the extra "raw materials" you eat will be used in milk production. Even malnourished women produce good quality milk. Their volume of milk may be slightly lower, however, and lactation will ultimately deplete the maternal stores of nutrients in order to supply the necessary components of milk. So, a poorly nourished mother's health would suffer before the quality of her milk would deteriorate. It is a rare American woman, however, who is so poorly nourished that this should concern her.

What You Need

Protein. The amount of milk you produce appears to be related to the amount of protein in your diet. An adequate intake of protein is therefore an obvious dietary goal. When pregnant, your protein need is 100 grams a day, but the Committee on Recommended Dietary Allowances of the Food and Nutrition Board recommends increasing your non-pregnancy protein intake of 46 grams to 66 grams a day during lactation.

Protein Sources

A peanut butter sandwich and a glass of milk (8 oz.)	20 gram
Cottage cheese (1/2 cup) and dried apricots (1/2 cup)	20 grams
Almonds (1/2 cup) and cheese (1 oz.)	20 grams
Two eggs and two biscuits	18 grams
Tuna, canned (3 oz.)	25 grams

Calcium. A well-balanced diet that includes some good sources of calcium is also important. When you are breastfeeding, you need about 2000 mg of calcium per day—at least 50 percent more than you need when you are not nursing. If this extra calcium is not freely available for your breast milk, it will be drawn out of your bones for milk production.

Calcium Sources

Almonds (1/2 cup)	165 mg
Soybeans, cooked (1 cup)	130 mg
Sesame seeds, whole (1 Tbs.)	105 mg
Swiss cheese (1 oz.)	260 mg
Cottage cheese (1 cup)	230 mg
Yogurt (8 oz.)	270 mg
Salmon, canned (3 oz.)	160 mg
Sardines, canned (3 oz.)	367 mg

Fluids. How much you drink should be regulated by your thirst. Although a low intake of fluids would not lead to a lower volume of milk, as was once thought, it can decrease your output of urine and lead to constipation. Do not go overboard on fluids, however, and think that you need to drink even when you are not thirsty. Some studies have indicated that excessive fluid intake can actually reduce the amount of milk you produce.

Vitamin Supplements. A vitamin supplement is a good idea for a breastfeeding mother. You cannot be sure that you will eat right every day, and your energy needs are higher when you are caring for a baby or small children. Many breastfeeding women find that a vitamin supplement, especially a vitamin B complex, helps them feel better and more energetic.

When you are taking a supplement, keep the following points in mind. Some young babies will experience digestive upset if their mothers consume iron supplements. If your supplement seems to upset your baby, try one without iron. Another concern is that some women are very sensitive to vitamin B_6 in amounts exceeding 50 to 100 mg a day. These very large doses can suppress lactation. If you take large doses, and you notice a dip in your milk supply, cut back on your intake of B_6.

What You Probably Do Not Need

• Many women believe that they need a large amount of cow's milk in order to produce human milk. Although milk is a good source of protein and calcium, it is not the only source. If you dislike milk or have an intolerance to it, try other sources of protein and calcium for your diet.

• There are also other sources of protein besides meat. Too much meat in the diet is probably more detrimental than helpful to your health.

• You may hear that you need beer to help your milk production or that any type of alcohol will aid your let-down reflex. But beer is not essential (or even helpful) to milk production. And although a small amount of alcohol can be relaxing, larger amounts can actually inhibit your let-down of milk. Also keep in mind that to some extent alcohol does pass through your milk to the baby.

• Brewer's yeast is often touted for its magical milk-making properties. The B vitamin content may aid milk production somewhat, but it is not essential.

Foods To Avoid

• **Lots of sugar.** Some mothers find that too much sugar gives their babies gas. Sugar can also deplete your natural antibodies, and it also robs your system of B vitamins during digestion, leaving you feeling tired.

• **Foods that contain chemical additives.** Since we are not sure to what extent these chemicals go through milk or what effect they may have on an infant, the safest approach is to avoid them as much as possible.

• **Onions.** Consuming onions can change the flavor of breast milk, and some babies object to it. Eliminate onions only if your baby seems to resist nursing after you have eaten them.

• **Spicy foods.** Some babies may have a problem with spicy foods, but most will not, so do not alter your diet unless you notice a problem in your baby. (See Colic, page 116)

Most babies do not react to the foods you eat. But if your baby experiences some digestive upset, and you suspect it may be something you are eating, consult the section on colic on pages 116 to 118 (Chapter 7), where we list some common offenders like milk, broccoli and cabbage.

Weight-Loss Diets While Nursing

Breastfeeding itself is a weight-reduction process. It has been found that some breastfeeding mothers will eat as many as 700 calories more per day than bottlefeeding mothers and still lose weight. Each day you use up fat resources that were laid down during pregnancy.

Losing weight while breastfeeding is a gradual, not an overnight, process, however. Do not despair if after three to five months you are not as slim as you would like to be. If at the end of a year (with no calorie or eating restrictions), you still are not at a satisfactory weight, you might consider a more aggressive approach to weight loss. Many women, however, lose their excess weight long before the year's end.

If you do decide to consciously try to lose weight, beware of rapid weight-loss methods. A weight loss of even a pound a week could lead to the release of formerly fat-bound toxins. Since these toxins go into your bloodstream and thus into your milk, your baby will ingest these undesirable substances.

If you feel strongly about losing weight more quickly, here are some sensible suggestions to help speed up the process.

• Eliminate empty calorie foods (like potato chips, soda pop and pretzels) from your diet.

• Cut out desserts and other sources of sugar; they add nothing to your health or your breast milk.

• If these measures are not enough, cut out the extra 300 to 500 calories you have been consuming for milk production.

This is one period of your life when you should not be overly concerned about your weight. Your energy needs are high, and if you do not eat to satisfy your hunger, you may find yourself tired and irritable. There will always be time for losing weight when your baby is older.

Exercise

An often overlooked need in a new mother's life is exercise. The benefits of exercise are always extensive, but at this time in your life they may be especially important.

Exercise helps

- control your weight
- reduce your body fat
- firm your muscles
- improve your digestion
- improve your circulation for better cardiovascular health
- provide an opportunity to meet people
- regulate your appetite
- provide release from emotional stress by increasing your energy and keeping you feeling alert

Demands on your time and energy are very real, but if you make exercise a priority, you should be able to find time for some physical activity. Simply getting out with the baby and going for a daily walk can be wonderful. Enrolling in an exercise class where you can bring your baby or organizing an exercise group with neighborhood friends are some other possibilities.

Back Pain

Exercise can also alleviate back pain, a problem that is especially common among breastfeeding mothers. This pain probably has several causes:

- The back stress from your recent pregnancy.
- The increased weight of your breasts (the breast of an average nonpregnant woman weighs about 200 grams; the breast of an average pregnant woman weighs about 400 to 600 grams; the breast of an average lactating woman weighs about 600 to 800 grams).
- The extra stress of holding and carrying your infant.
- Nursing (improperly) in a hunched-over and unsupported position, typically described as a "round-shouldered posture."

Given all of these influences, it is no wonder that new mothers have backaches. A closer look at the supporting structure of the breast will show us what type of support a new mother's body provides and how exercises will relieve her discomfort. The following material and exercises were developed with the specific needs of the breastfeeding mother in mind by Dr. Georgann Marx, a Denver chiropractor and director of Back Health Institute.

Breast Anatomy

The breast consists of glandular tissue, fat cells and connective tissue called suspensory ligaments. Ligaments play the major role in supporting the breast, since it contains no muscles itself and muscle tone contributes only minimally to breast support. However, since the breast is attached to and sits on top of muscle, toning these muscles can indirectly provide added support.

The first place a new breastfeeding woman feels stress is in the back muscles, which provide the extra support needed when she nurses in the "round-shouldered" position. Additionally, the "round-shouldered" position overactivates the pectoralis minor muscle, the muscle that is attached to the front of the shoulder and fans down to the third, fourth and fifth ribs in the direction of the nipple. Overusing this muscle strains the area below the collar bone.

Overusing the pectoralis muscle also creates an imbalance with the muscles in the back that are not being worked as hard as this front muscle. When this happens, the breastfeeding mother will experience aching muscular discomfort between her shoulder blades, at the top of her shoulders and at the base of her neck.

To relieve this discomfort, a breastfeeding mother needs both to stretch the overused pectoralis minor muscle and to strengthen the weak upper back muscles. The following groups of exercises help accomplish this. They consist of a stretch and strengthening technique. These exercises are recommended even if your back does not hurt, since they will help you maintain good posture and increase your energy level. If you *do* have back pain, do at least the minimum, but feel free to do more if you like.

Do these exercises once a day; they will take about five minutes. Repeat each exercise five times and hold each exercise position for five seconds. Increase repetition as you are able.

Exercise 1. Go to an open doorway. Interlock your hands behind your head, then press your elbow against the doorway. Keep your heels flat on the floor and lean straight forward (do not bend at the waist) until you feel the stretch under your arm. Perform this exercise on both arms.

Exercise 2. Sit or stand and interlock your hands behind your head, but do not exert pressure on your head with your hands. Force your elbows back and imagine that you are touching your shoulder blades together. You should feel your muscles pulling between your shoulders.

Exercise 3. This exercise can be done either sitting or standing. Clasp your hands together behind your back and lift your hands upward about ten inches or until you feel the pull. Keep your back straight. You will feel the pulling in your upper arms and the stretching between your shoulder blades.

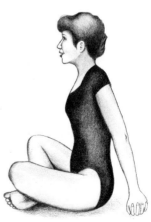

Exercise 4. During this three-part exercise, you will need to sit in a cross-legged position. The purpose of this series is to strengthen your upper back.

Part A 1. Raise your arms to shoulder level at your sides and bring your forearms forward to a 90 degree angle. Keep your palms and forearms parallel to the floor.

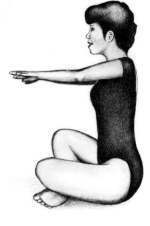

2. Pull your elbows back and hold.

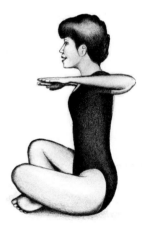

Part B 1. Bend your elbows at a 90 degree angle with your forearms pointing up and palms forward. Keep your forearms parallel to the wall.

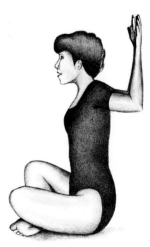

2. Pull your elbows back and hold.

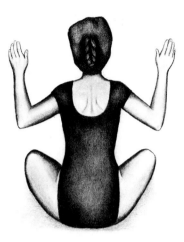

Part C   1. Bend your elbows, bringing your forearms parallel to your sides with your forearms and hands pointing down and your palms facing back.

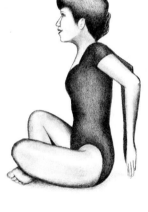

2. Pull your elbows back and hold.

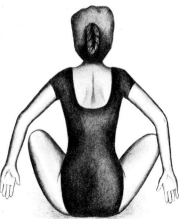

Exercise 5. Sit in a cross-legged position and circle one shoulder up and forward while the other shoulder circles down and back and alternate in a figure eight pattern. Do this continuously and do not hold any position. You will alternately feel both stretching and strengthening in your upper back and the muscles on your chest wall above your breasts.

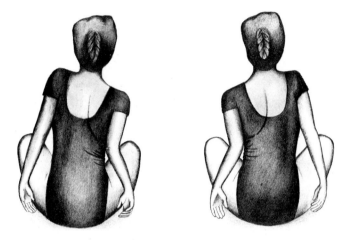

Exercise 6. 1. Lie face down on the floor and rest your chin on the floor, hands above your head.

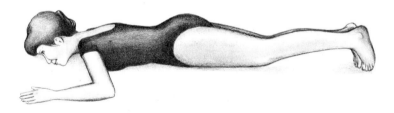

2. Elevate your hands, arms and shoulders. Keep your elbows and wrists parallel to the floor and your feet on the floor. You will feel stretching in your mid-lower back.

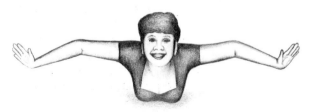

Exercise 7. Lie on your back on the floor with your knees up and your hands placed about ten inches from your sides. Press your elbows and hands into the floor. Your shoulder blades and upper back will go up, but your head should remain on the floor. You will feel this exercise down your sides and in your shoulders.

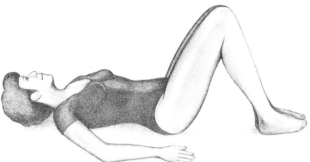

Exercise 8.
Part A

1. Stand facing the inside corner of two walls (or an open doorway). Place your feet approximately one comfortable step away from the corner or doorway. Put one of your hands against each wall, with your elbows straight and your arms at shoulder height.

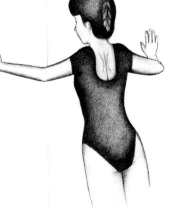

2. Allow your body to slowly move into the corner or doorway as you bend your elbows. Keep your heels flat on the floor, your spine and knees straight, and your abdomen firm. Don't let your hips sag forward. Hold in this position for five seconds and then slowly push out. This exercise will strengthen the middle of your back and the back of your arms.

Part B   1. Use the same position as
above, but raise your hands
so they are even with your
head.

2. Repeat the same motion as
in Part A. This part of the
exercise will strengthen your
mid-lower back and the back
of your arms.

Part C   1. Use the same position as
above, but lower your hands
to your waist level.

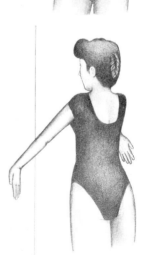

2. Repeat same motion as in Part A. In this part you will be strengthening your upper-mid back and the back of your arms.

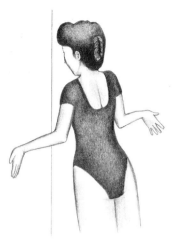

Clothing for the Nursing Mother

Once your baby is born, you will find that in addition to wanting to feel attractive and comfortable, you will also need a somewhat specialized wardrobe.

Nursing Bras

A nursing bra differs from a regular bra in that without removing the bra, you can open the cups like flaps to make your breasts available to your baby. Although nursing bras are not absolutely essential, they are preferred by most nursing mothers. Here are the features to consider when purchasing a nursing bra.

Size. If you shop for your nursing bras while you are still pregnant, remember to buy a nursing bra that is both a size and a cup size larger than the bra you are wearing during pregnancy, and only buy one nursing bra before your baby is born. After you are home from the hospital and you are nursing, you will have a more accurate idea of your size.

Fabric. The best fabric is 100 percent cotton since it will let your skin breathe. Synthetic fabrics hold in moisture, which can lead to sore nipples. Some nursing bras are made of cotton but have a synthetic liner or padding. Simply cut out the liner or padding and you will have an all-cotton bra.

The Fastener. You will find that cups on nursing bras can be fastened by snaps, latches or velcro. Velcro or snaps allow you to open and close your bra with one hand, which is quite useful. With velcro, however, everyone in your presence can hear each time you open your bra, and the texture of velcro may irritate your skin.

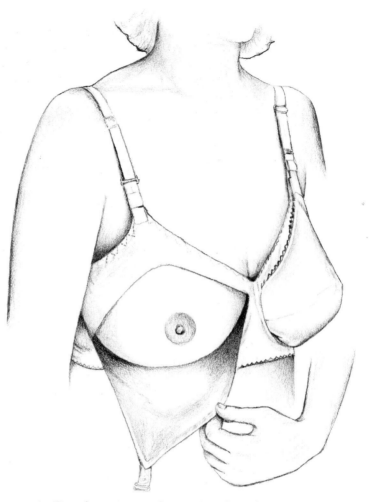

Nursing Bra

Allows you to open the cups like flaps to make your breast easily available to your baby.

Support. Try the nursing bra on and make sure it supports you adequately. During the latter part of your pregnancy, your breasts will be quite large, so you should be able to evaluate the support the bra offers.

Straps. Because of the increased weight of your breasts, straps that are fairly wide will be more comfortable than narrow straps. Some women prefer elastic straps, and although it is rare to find them in a nursing bra, you can buy elastic and insert a piece yourself.

Other Tips • Another possibility, especially once you are past the early, very full weeks of nursing, is simply to use a regular bra and pull up one side when you nurse. A non-nursing bra is less expensive and sometimes more comfortable. You cannot do this with an underwire bra, however, and a regular bra may not work for you if you have very large breasts.

• Some women report great comfort, support and convenience from athletic bras, which are often 100 percent cotton and all elasticized, so they are easy to pull up for nursing. They also offer a great deal of comfortable support because the straps cross in back.

• A "sleeping bra" can be wonderful for night wear if you are leaking in the early weeks, since it allows you to wear nursing pads and still be comfortable. Later, you may find that the lightness and elasticity of a sleeping bra make it a good nursing bra, too.

Convenient and Discreet Clothing

While you are nursing, you will find that two-piece outfits offer the most convenient and discreet way to nurse. Wear a slightly loose shirt or blouse that you can pull up when you nurse (rather than unbutton); the baby covers the bottom half of your breast and the blouse covers the top.

When you are getting dressed up, wear two-piece outfits that make nursing easy. A dress with a zipper down the back just will not work. Some women like "nursing fashions"—a dress or blouse with slits down both sides of the front that are usually fastened with velcro and often disguised with ruffles or pleats. This design offers another approach to convenient and discreet nursing.

Postpartum Clothes

After your baby is born, you may be disappointed to discover that those pre-pregnancy clothes you longed to wear again still do not fit. During this phase, when your body is gradually resuming its former shape, it is hard to find appropriate clothes to wear. You do not want to wear your maternity clothes anymore, and you hate to buy all new clothes in a larger size for this temporary period.

One way to feel more attractive and less depressed about your postpartum body is to wear wrap-around skirts. They do not look like maternity clothes, they will surely fit, and each week you can just tie them a little tighter. You will feel as though you are wearing "normal" clothes, and you will be able to nurse conveniently since you can simply pull up your blouse.

Equipment for the Nursing Mother

Many experienced breastfeeding mothers find that they can get by with much less "essential equipment" than the baby magazines recommend. Before you buy any nursing equipment, look closely at your specific needs.

Nursing Pads

Virtually every new nursing mother needs nursing pads—circular pieces of absorbent paper material or cloth that are worn inside your bra cup to absorb leaking milk. Try several types—there are some variations in shape, material and price—and decide which you like the best.

Disposable Nursing Pads. Available in most pharmacies. Avoid plastic-lined pads, which hold in moisture and contribute to sore nipples.

Reusable Nursing Pads. Can be made at home by cutting diapers or old cotton T-shirts into circles and then sewing several layers together. You may also be able to buy these, and although they are initially more expensive than disposables, you can wash and reuse them, so they will not cost more in the long run. The Happy Family Products Co. is one source of reusable nursing pads. You will need quite a few pairs since they must be changed frequently.

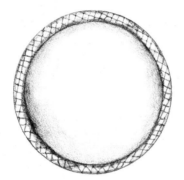

Disposable Nursing Pads
Available in most pharmacies. Avoid plastic-lined pads which hold in moisture and contribute to sore nipples.

Reusable Nursing Pads
Can be washed and reused. You can buy them or make them at home by cutting up diapers into circles and then sewing several layers together.

Breast Pumps

Cylinder Pump. If you need a breast pump, we recommend the cylinder-type hand-held pump. It works with a piston-like motion, is very effective, can be sterilized conveniently in the dishwasher and is small enough to be carried in your purse. There are many similar brands on the market.

Bicycle-Horn Pump. Although the bicycle-horn hand pump is the least expensive type on the market, we discourage its use. It is not very effective, and it is usually painful to use.

Electric Pump. If you are a nursing mother who works outside the home, you might consider buying a small electric pump. Two such pumps are the AXi-Care CM4 and the Mary Jane Electric Pump.

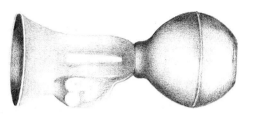

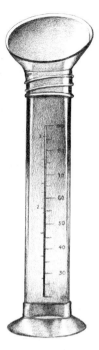

Breast Pumps

Bicycle Pump

The bicycle-horn hand pump is the least expensive type. However, we discourage its use because it is not effective and is often painful.

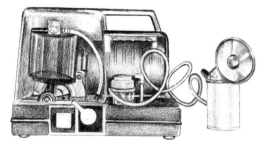

Cylinder Pump

The cylinder-type hand-held pump is recommended. It is very effective, can be sterilized in the dishwasher, and is small enough to carry in your purse.

Electric Pump

If you are a nursing mother that works, consider buying an electric pump. You can rent a full-sized pump as shown above, or purchase a smaller model. Two effective models are the Axi-Care (CM4) and the Mary Jane Electric Pump.

Rubber-Lined Pads

If you find it easier to nurse your baby in bed at night, put a large rubber pad under your baby to protect your sheets. You can buy rubber-lined pads in different sizes, or you can buy the material by the yard at some fabric stores and cut it to size.

A Baby Frontpack

It is a rare nursing mother who does not feel that a front baby carrier is indispensable. The straps of a baby pack cross in the back, so your baby's weight is more evenly distributed than it would be if you were carrying the baby in your arms, and that means less strain on your back. A frontpack will also free your hands, and many models, like the McPack and the Snuggli, allow your baby to nurse while in the pack.

Your Rest and Sleep Levels

In terms of your own level of energy, the first problem you face with a new baby may be matching the reality of the experience with your expectations of what it would be like.

Your Expectations May Have Been

• When I quit work and am home full time, I will have more free time than I have ever had before.

• Babies sleep all the time.

• My baby will be sleeping through the night in a few weeks.

• I imagine my baby will nurse according to a schedule—probably about every four hours.

• Since I ate well and exercised during my pregnancy, I will be back to my old shape and activities right away.

The Reality Will More Likely Be

• You will feel as though you are suffering from terminal fatigue.

• Young babies sleep more lightly than older children and adults; during these periods they are likely to wake up for a feeding.

• You will develop a sleep pattern we call "punctuated sleep." Your body will adjust to feeling rested from several naps rather than one long stretch of sleep.

• Babies who have learned to trust their parents will express their very real night needs for food and contact. (These needs generally exist longer than "weeks.")

• Breastfed babies nurse often. We are a "continuous contact mammal" with a low protein milk and frequent nursing needs.

• Many babies just do not need a great deal of sleep.

Like marriage, parenthood is a permanent change. Your "old normal" will never be "normal" for you again. But like marriage, parenthood can enhance your life, and the adjustments are well worth it.

How to Survive

• Put it in perspective. This is a brief period. There will be a time when sleep will not be the most interesting subject in your life.

• Nap when your baby naps.

• Resist doing all those household jobs you have been planning to do in the evening and go to bed early instead.

• Do whatever relaxes you. Some women use Transcendental Meditation or another kind of meditation. Women who also have a toddler might try lying on the couch during "Sesame Street." For some, taking long nursing breaks in bed is enough. Also, hiring a teenager to come in for an hour or two in the afternoon to play with the baby while you rest can be a wonderful relief.

We promise, one day you will be awake for the evening news again!

Your Activity Level

At first, you will need to temporarily cut back on your activities because of your energy and time limitations. Recognize that mothering is full-time work, and that you will have very little time for yourself. For your mental health, try to give yourself something special every day. Get some quiet time to read the paper, take a peaceful bath, have an occasional lunch out or go to bridge club or a discussion group. Learn to set priorities. There are no supermoms, so accept your limitations and do not chastise yourself. Give yourself credit for the good job you are doing.

The following guidelines may help you form some realistic expectations about what you will be able to do after the birth of your baby.

Week 1. Do nothing except lie in bed, rest and nurse your baby. Keep visitors to a minimum so you do not become overtired from playing hostess. Try to limit them to family and your closest friends.

Week 2. Continue to rest and take it easy, but you can take on some of the household work. Keep visits very brief.

Weeks 3-6. Gradually increase your share of the household work, and start to resume some social activities. At this point you will enjoy guests and the chance to show off your beautiful new baby.

Weeks 7-12. Begin some type of exercise you like. You and your baby will enjoy social outings.

From Three Months On. Work back up to your normal level of activity, although your activities may be different than they once were.

Drugs and Medications in Breast Milk

Drug and medication safety should concern everyone since, as one toxicologist has said, "Every drug is a controlled poison." The issue is doubly important, however, for the breastfeeding woman. Everything you ingest now must also be screened for your baby. This added responsibility requires some awareness and caution.

Questions to Consider

You should ask a number of questions about any drug you consider taking:

• **Will the drug go from my bloodstream into my breast milk?** Most drugs you take will be present to some extent in your milk. The factors affecting how much of the drug will be present are many and complex, and include variables such as the fat solubility of the drug and the composition of your breast milk. Some drugs are present in breast milk in concentrations at or above the level present in the mother's blood; other drugs do not appear at all or in trace amounts only.

• **If the drug is present in my breast milk, will it harm my baby?** Your chief guideline here is that if you would not possibly give the medication directly to an infant, you must question its safety.

• **Is it possible to sensitize my baby to the drug?** An example of this type of concern would be penicillin.

• **If my infant is already taking another medication, how safely will the two drugs interact?**

Resources to Use

If you are planning to take any medication (either prescription or over-the-counter), you need to check with a knowledgeable source to get answers to these questions about its safety. The following list cites some good resources on drugs and breast milk:

• Call the La Leche League. They have a drug list which lists most drugs, their safety or danger level, and medical sources for the research.

• Ask your health-care professional, but only if he or she is knowledgeable and supportive of breastfeeding. Unfortunately, some medical professionals will tell a breastfeeding mother to wean if she is taking any medication because they are not well informed about the safety of the drug and think weaning is the safest approach. Do not casually wean your baby over a medication. It is your right (and responsibility) to seek a second opinion.

• Call a pharmacist if you need a good recommendation for an alternate drug.

• If your city has a drug hotline, call it and ask for the information you need.

• Check the publications that exist on the subject.

Over-the-Counter Drugs

Many common over-the-counter drugs have been taken by breastfeeding mothers with no known harmful effects. Do not take any medications casually, but if you really need relief, the following nonprescription preparations are probably safe for a breastfeeding mother to use.

Analgesics
Excedrin
Tylenol
Aspirin
Bufferin
Cope

Antacid
Maalox
Mylanta
Titrilac

Antihistamines
Triaminic
Contac
Sudafed
Sinutabs

Laxatives
Castor Oil
Senna
Magnesia

Do not overlook natural remedies for your health problem. A natural remedy may take a little more research and effort, but it could be quite worthwhile. For example, headache sufferers often find relief from a neck massage, a long steamy bath and a cup of very hot tea. If you have a cold, try taking extra vitamin C, running a vaporizer, resting, drinking plenty of fluids, eating chicken soup and drinking licorice or anise tea.

Drugs in Everyday Life

We would like to offer some additional information on "drugs" that may be part of your daily life and may be overlooked when you think of breastfeeding safety.

Caffeine. Only a small amount of the caffeine you consume actually goes through the milk. In fact, the level in a mother's milk is only one percent of the level in her blood. So if you consume a moderate amount of caffeine, usually no effect is seen in the infant. But caffeine *does* accumulate in an infant's system (smoking increases the effect of caffeine, too). As a result, if you consume a fairly large amount of caffeine—the equivalent of six to eight cups of coffee per day—over time you may see some irritability and sleeplessness in your baby. Some babies do not seem to be affected by moderate caffeine intake while others are quite sensitive to it. If you cut down or eliminate your caffeine consumption (and remember that many carbonated drinks, tea, some medications and chocolate also contain caffeine), it will take about a week for the effect on the baby to disappear.

Alcohol. Light to moderate alcohol use (one or two drinks in a day) will not be a problem for the breastfeeding mother and her infant. Alcohol in greater amounts poses a problem because it can suppress the release of oxytocin from the pituitary gland, interfering with the let-down reflex. Babies of heavy drinkers will probably get less milk and be sleepy as a result of the alcohol they ingest through the milk. In addition to possible drowsiness and even deep sleep, these infants may also gain less weight and grow less than they would have.

Nicotine. Nicotine in breast milk can be a serious problem for an infant. If you smoke a pack of cigarettes a day, your baby will receive about 10 percent of the minimum lethal dose of nicotine; two packs a day constitutes 20 percent, and so on. If you are a heavy smoker (20 to 30 cigarettes a day), your baby may experience nausea, vomiting, abdominal cramps and diarrhea. Smoking is also known to interfere with the let-down reflex.

Secondhand smoke is a major problem for babies, too. It is fairly common for babies to exhibit an allergic reaction to the gases released by a burning cigarette. Babies exposed to secondhand smoke also suffer from more pneumonia and bronchitis.

Marijuana. For several reasons, smoking marijuana is not advisable for breastfeeding mothers. Animal experiments show that the amount of marijuana that comes through breast milk is enough to cause structural changes in the brain cells of the nursling. Also, lower levels of prolactin are found in mothers who smoke marijuana, so it can be assumed that their ability to produce milk would be at least somewhat impaired. The other possible dangers stemming from this practice include secondhand smoke, the mother's impaired judgment, and her decreased ability to care for her infant.

Your Reproductive System

Your Menstrual Cycle

One of the many pleasant effects of nursing is the absence of monthly periods, a condition called *lactation amenorrhea.* Menstruation is suppressed because the predominance of prolactin during nursing prevents ovulation. In order for ovulation to be suppressed, however, your infant must nurse frequently and without restriction or your periods may return. For example, if your baby starts solids, starts sleeping through the night, uses a pacifier for her comfort sucking, or even misses some feedings, your hormonal balance may shift and your menstrual cycles *may* resume.

There is a great deal of individual variation in when a nursing mother's periods will return. Occasionally a woman's period may start within a month or two after childbirth. At the other extreme is the woman whose periods do not resume until several months after her baby weans. The typical range for a woman who practices unrestricted nursing is from seven to fifteen months of amenorrhea.

The effects of the resumption of menstrual periods are not significant. Many women report some tenderness in their breasts during their periods. Some women feel that they have slightly less milk during their periods. This is nothing to be concerned about; there will still be enough for the baby during this very brief dip in supply.

Contraception　Many women assume that the return of their menstrual periods also means the return of fertility, but the relationship between the two processes is not that clear-cut. You may ovulate prior to that first period, after it or, even more typically, one or two months later.

Breastfeeding, in fact, is not an entirely reliable form of contraception by itself. The risk of conceiving during a period of demand nursing without contraception is five percent, which is higher than many women are willing to take. Some additional form of contraception is recommended if you do not want to take that risk. Most forms of birth control will not present any special problem for the breastfeeding woman. Recommended methods include the diaphragm, cervical cap, condom, vaginal suppository, cream or jelly, or a vaginal sponge.

The use of any birth control pill is contraindicated for breast-feeding women. The hormones in birth control pills will decrease your milk supply and lower its protein, fat, lactose, calcium and phosphorus content. The hormones also pass through your milk to the baby and can result in the abnormal enlargement of an infant's breasts. A hormone-coated IUD would pose the same threat.

Some health-care professionals may try to reassure you of the safety of the "mini-pill," which contains only progesterone, by telling you that it has a lower dose of hormones and that no harmful effects have been seen as a result of its use. If you feel so strongly about the use of the birth control pill that you would be willing to wean your baby if you could not use it, then you might go ahead and take the "mini-pill" because it is probably less harmful than either a new pregnancy or switching your baby to formula. But if you are willing to use another form of contraception, it would be far better to explore those possibilities instead.

Another caution worth mentioning concerns the IUD. Although IUDs have been used successfully by many breastfeeding women, they are more likely to perforate the uterus of a lactating woman, because of the uterine contractions that accompany nursing, especially during the first few months when the uterus is still involuting. If you strongly prefer the IUD as a method of birth control, you might consider using another form during the first two months and then having your IUD inserted.

If you have reasons for wanting to use breastfeeding as a natural method of birth control, you will need to inform yourself about the details of this system. Read John and Sheila Kipley's *The Art of Natural Family Planning.* There is also an organization that offers instruction on this and other methods of natural birth control called The Couple to Couple League.

Becoming Pregnant

If you *do* become pregnant while you are breastfeeding, it will affect nursing, but it does not necessitate weaning. Your breasts and nipples may be tender, your milk supply will gradually diminish, and eventually it will turn to colostrum. At that point, many breastfeeding babies will wean themselves because of the lower volume and changed taste of the milk. A baby who still has a strong need to nurse, however, may continue to nurse in spite of these changes. Do not worry about this. Since colostrum does not come in a finite quantity, you cannot "use it up" by nursing one baby while carrying another. You will continue to produce colostrum until several days after your new baby is born.

Many mothers are concerned that they may be robbing the fetus of nourishment by nursing their baby. This is not the case. The small amount of colostrum you produce will not be a drain on the nutrients going to the fetus. However, you will notice your own increased hunger and additional need for sleep.

Sexuality and the Breastfeeding Woman

How breastfeeding will affect your sex drive is a somewhat complicated question. Many nursing women will notice that their sex drive seems to diminish, but this may be due less to breastfeeding than to the demands of motherhood. Some factors, however, are related to breastfeeding.

Lower Estrogen Levels. Because it suppresses ovulation, nursing keeps estrogen levels lower longer. This may contribute somewhat to a weakened sex drive, but it is certainly not the most dominant factor. If it were, all nursing women would have the same response. Lower estrogen levels might cause a woman's sexual response to take longer, but it will not prevent it entirely. In reality, the factors that follow have a greater effect.

Exhaustion. Exhaustion in either sex, at any stage of life, is extremely detrimental to sex drive. One solution would be to make love in the morning, afternoon or early evening if possible.

The Touched-Out Syndrome. By the end of the day many new nursing mothers have had so much physical closeness, cuddling, stroking and holding with their babies that their need for physical contact has already been greatly satisfied.

Total Absorption. It is completely natural for a new mother to be so interested in her new baby that she excludes everything else. It is very helpful if the father's energies are directed toward his fascination with his new baby, rather than his feelings of competition (see more on this in Chapter 6).

Differing Needs. A woman needs to adjust to and enjoy her baby, to nurse her and to focus on her. She also has an intense need for sleep. Her partner's needs are different, however; he may need reassurance that their status as a couple is not threatened.

Pain. If you had a fairly large episiotomy or tear, intercourse can be extremely painful for a surprisingly long time. Try to position yourself on top during intercourse so you can have more control over penetration and movement. Patience and gentleness will also help a great deal. Another suggestion for a painful episiotomy is to use comfrey tea. Throw three tea bags into your sitz bath, or wrap the leaves, which have been soaked in hot water, in some gauze and place this "pack" against your perineum. Your sanitary napkin will hold it in place.

Vaginal Dryness. Because your hormonal state is different, a lactating woman will have less natural lubrication in her vagina during sex. Using a lubricant such as K-Y jelly will solve this problem. Avoid hormone creams or products containing petroleum. Petroleum products can deteriorate rubber and affect certain types of contraceptive devices, like diaphragms.

Leaking. Because the "let-down" hormone, oxytocin, is also released during sex, a nursing woman may find that she leaks milk during lovemaking. Most couples do not find this at all disturbing, but a few are uncomfortable with it.

Embarrassment and Fear. Many new mothers do not feel good about their postpartum bodies, which may prevent them from feeling as "sexy" as they once did. In addition, they may fear becoming pregnant again.

Lower Nipple Sensitivity. If you enjoy nipple stimulation during lovemaking, you may notice some diminished response temporarily during the period you are nursing.

Baby's Radar. In the early months of life, a baby and her mother seem to sleep in closely tuned patterns. So when the mother becomes stimulated, the baby may very well wake up because she senses it. This effect goes away fairly soon and is certainly not in operation all the time.

As a couple, you will need some extra patience and understanding during the first few months after the birth of your baby. Your relationship will normalize. All you need is a little time.

Your Support System

If this is your first baby, you are probably home during the day for the first time. Although you have looked forward to this time and it is wonderful in many ways, you may find yourself feeling lonely and isolated at times. In order to make this the best time it can be for you, you may need to create a support system for yourself.

Friends You cannot underestimate your need for adult company. Although your baby is a great source of pleasure for you, you will begin to crave an adult conversation. Your old friends may still be at the workplace you left and unavailable during the day. You will be happiest if you make an effort to meet some other young parents who are home with their babies, too. Take walks, go to your neighborhood park or take parenting classes. Being able to share with other women who are interested and involved with babies makes motherhood more fun.

Support Organizations Organizations are another good source of support for you. La Leche League (LLL) offers information, encouragement and support to breastfeeding mothers. The groups are organized on a neighborhood basis, so joining La Leche League is also a good way to meet mothers of breastfeeding babies in your area. Each group has at least one certified Leader, who leads the discussions at the monthly meetings, can answer questions on any aspect of breastfeeding and is available for telephone help.

La Leche League is a volunteer organization that has optional (but much appreciated) annual dues. Dues-paying members receive a bimonthly newsletter. Women attending La Leche League meetings can check out books from the group's library, take reprints on a wide variety of topics and receive help for any type of breastfeeding problem. The atmosphere within most LLL groups is very open and accepting.

If there is no LLL in your area or if you have special needs, it may be worthwhile to form your own support group. Women have formed their own mothers of twins, working/nursing mothers and mothers of adopted children groups, for example. You may also be able to make a support group of neighborhood friends.

Social Groups

Belonging to or even forming social groups can be a great boost to your suddenly altered social life. You might seek social contact from a book discussion group or a bridge club. Or you might prefer a group that is purely social. Many new parents change the focus of their social lives from "going out" to either having friends over for supper or going to their friends' homes for a meal.

Some couples even form a "supper club" out of three or four couples who have children the same age as theirs. Each couple takes a turn making supper for the whole group. It can be planned on a weekly or monthly basis, and it provides a fun meal out, the company of people with similar interests, and no babysitting problems since the babies are naturally invited!

Support Yourself

During this special yet demanding time in your life, you may find yourself under a great deal of pressure from many sources. You can listen to all the well-meaning advice you hear and sort it out for yourself. The most important thing for you to remember, though, is to trust your own instincts. It is your baby, it is your lifestyle, and you need to make decisions that work for you.

Chapter Six The Nursing Family

The birth of your first baby will change your life in many ways. Some changes will be subtle, some more obvious, but you will feel them in every part of your life. Perhaps the most obvious is that instead of being a couple, you are now a family, and you will need to adjust to and become comfortable with the ways you function together as parents.

In this chapter, we will address the nursing family. Although the act of breastfeeding involves only the mother and baby, the

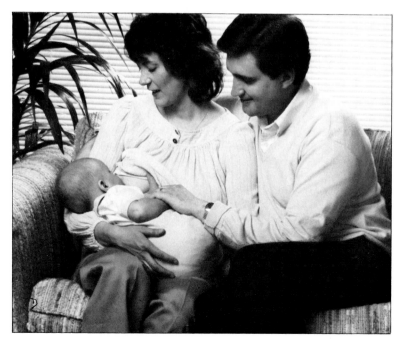

The birth of your first baby will change your life. You are now a family, instead of a couple. You need time to adjust to the way you function together as parents.

nursing relationship affects the whole family. And, of course, the entire family is involved in the nurturing of this new infant.

The Father

A father plays an indispensable role in the emotional and psychological development of his child. He is important to the formation of a strong, healthy family unit and will contribute to it in many ways as your family grows. Besides contributing to the child's feelings of security and being loved, he aids the development of the child's self-esteem and his sense of sexual identity. Also, if he is gone most of the day to work and then returns each evening—a new and yet familiar face—part of his irresistible appeal is his combined familiarity and novelty.

But in the beginning of the life of your baby and of your newly formed family, his major role (ideally) will be to nurture and support the breastfeeding relationship. Some people fear that breastfeeding excludes a father from parenting his baby. But there is more to parenting than feeding a baby. As an insightful father once said, "A truly creative father can think of more ways to show his love for his baby than to stick a bottle in his mouth." In the long run, the care the father gives is just as important as the mother's care. While the mother may command all the attention at first, as the baby becomes more alert and playful, the father's participation will grow, and it will continue to grow throughout the child's life.

Supporting the Breastfeeding Relationship

Since breastfeeding is central to the baby's well-being on every level, the most important gift a father can give his baby is the assurance that the nursing relationship will be protected and fostered. He can do this in many ways.

• He can offer support and encouragement to the breastfeeding mother. Compliments and expressions of pride, especially when they come from her partner, mean a great deal.

• He can shield his partner from criticism and nonsupportive comments. If the criticism comes from his family, he should be especially sure to assert that he shares and stands behind the decision to breastfeed.

• He can help make it possible for mother and baby to have a great deal of time together from the very first. Everyone will be happier with a calm and quiet beginning in which to adjust and learn all there is to learn. A father can also delay or limit visits from relatives and friends.

• If he can arrange to take vacation time or paternity leave from work when mother and baby come home from the hospital, he will give them a most wonderful gift. No one can

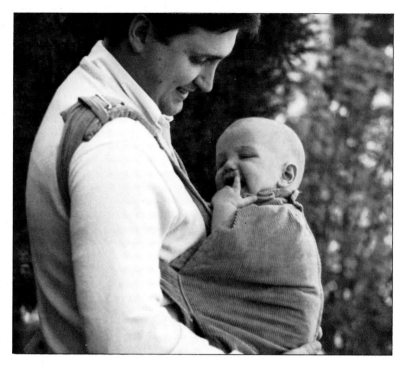

In order to feel close to your baby as his father, spend time getting to know him. Begin handling the baby as early as possible. The moment of birth is a good time to start.

help with the same competence as the baby's father. He alone is completely familiar with your house and its routines. This arrangement also enhances bonding between the father and baby, allows him to become competent with infant care, and gives everyone a chance to adjust to the new feeling of "familyhood."

• He can provide extra physical help, including shopping, cleaning, cooking, doing laundry, changing diapers, bathing the baby and so on. The extra work a new baby generates is just too much for one person.

• He can bring the baby in for night nursings, a service that is most appreciated by an overtired new mother.

Building the Father/Baby Relationship

In order to feel close to his baby, a father needs to spend time getting to know him. Since a new baby does not "play" yet, the major way to spend time with him is to "take care" of him. Some mothers, however, feel they are more competent at baby care, so they fail to encourage the father's involvement and participation in caretaking—a loss to all three.

Most fathers want to feel competent with baby care, and they do not have a monopoly on new-parent awkwardness; mothers feel exactly the same way. The only way to become comfortable with this new set of skills is to plunge in and start doing it. Begin handling the baby as early as possible; the moment of birth is a good time to start.

Fathers also need time to focus some physical attention on their babies. Physical contact is especially important, both because it aids the bonding process and because it makes the relationship more enjoyable. And, because they cannot nurse, fathers need to find their own ways to comfort their babies. Some comforting techniques used by many fathers include the following:

• Singing to a fussy baby will often calm and quiet him.

• Carrying the baby in a frontpack is usually an effective way to comfort a baby and put him to sleep.

• Walking or rocking a tired or cranky baby are time-tested methods which rarely fail to soothe.

• Even the most miserable baby is usually soothed by a car ride. Many fathers have been known to go for an evening "snooze cruise" with their colicky or teething baby and return with a sleeping one. Apparently the sound and vibration of the car's engine are comforting to the baby.

• Putting the baby in the stroller and going for a walk can also do wonders for a crying baby. The motion, sights and sounds must be distracting and allow the baby to refocus and become content.

Fathering a breastfed baby can be a satisfying and joyful experience. Most men glow with pride as they see their nursing newborn thrive and grow into a healthy, alert, beautiful baby.

Common Concerns of the Father

It is only natural that new parenthood should also bring some doubts and questions. Breastfeeding itself may raise some concerns in the minds of new fathers. Here are some common concerns that fathers express or questions they ask, followed by a discussion of each.

• **I feel uncomfortable about my wife exposing her breasts to nurse.** Most new fathers imagine that breastfeeding involves exposing the mother's breast to all who are present. Actually, it is very easy to nurse discreetly. (See page 60.)

• **Is it safe to bring a baby into bed to nurse? When will our baby begin sleeping through the night in his own bed?** Bringing the baby into bed is a safe and nurturing practice. You will not roll over on the baby; the same instinct that keeps you from falling off the bed will keep you from rolling onto your baby. Your baby will outgrow the need for contact during the night and will sleep independently in his own bed after he has fulfilled some of his dependency needs.

• **Will it spoil my child if my wife offers him the breast as soon as he whimpers?** On the contrary, giving your baby too much love cannot spoil him. The concept of spoiling should never be applied to infancy. Satisfying his early needs for food, closeness and security will allow your baby to grow into a trusting and independent child.

• **Should we let our baby wean himself from the breast? What if he never weans?** Children who have had their dependency needs satisfied, as a self-weaned baby would have, become *more* independent, not less. Also, there are immunological and nutritional benefits to longer nursing that have only recently come to light. The far-reaching benefits of baby-led weaning are discussed in greater detail in Chapter 9, "As Your Baby Grows Older."

• **Will my wife's breastfeeding affect our sex life?** A couple's sex life might be a little more low key in the early months of new parenthood, due to the exhaustion this period brings, not to breastfeeding. Nursing will cause vaginal dryness, however, but this can be easily managed by using a lubricant such as K-Y jelly. Also, some men feel unsure about breast stimulation during lovemaking. They wonder if their wive's breasts are reserved only for the baby during this period. The answer to this depends, of course, on the woman's feelings about breast stimulation. But as long as she is comfortable with it, there is no reason not to include this practice in your lovemaking. The breasts serve two biological purposes; they are both mammary glands and erogenous zones, and one role need not exclude the other. For a more detailed discussion of this subject, see page 87.

• **Will having a baby threaten our relationship?** Your relationship as a couple should remain stable and intact, especially once your baby is a little older. Although you are now a family as well, make an effort to keep the special "couple" feeling between you strong. Breastfeeding babies do not tie you down; as a matter of fact, they are extremely portable. Do not change your lifestyle if you enjoy going out. Throw a diaper in the car and go. Most babies enjoy car rides and the noise and stimulation of new places and faces. Eating out and going to a movie are ideal outings for a breastfed baby, since it is easy to nurse in a dim booth or dark theater.

During the early months of new parenthood, a father needs to be prepared for his partner to focus on the baby. This should be accepted as normal. The mother's interest in the baby is natural and does not mean she loves her partner any less. As a father, he will probably find that he, too, is quite absorbed by this fascinating new addition to his life.

A man will find that fathering his breastfeeding baby and supporting his breastfeeding partner will be easier and more rewarding if he is convinced of the value of breastfeeding. He can educate himself by reading, attending classes or encouraging his partner to share what she has learned about nursing. At the same time, the more obvious advantages of breastfeeding should be told to the father. The nonexistent formula bills have to be appreciated, as does the ease of satisfying the baby's needs. Most of all, fathers appreciate the pride they feel knowing that their child is receiving the very best.

Siblings of the Breastfed Baby

If this is not your first baby, you probably worried during your pregnancy about how you could ever love your new baby as much as you love your first child. This is a common worry. The mother-love you experience with your first baby is a new height of love, and you may feel it can never be duplicated, only diluted by the presence of a new child. But when your new child is born, you will be adding love to love and that just makes more love. You will discover a whole new source of unlimited love, and your previous concern will vanish.

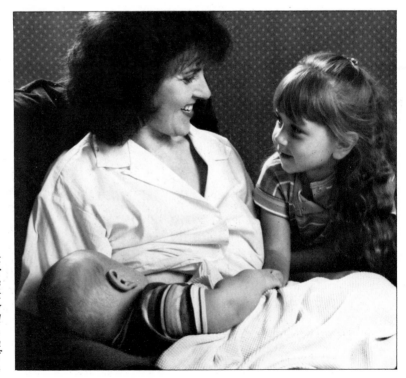

You may worry that you cannot love your new baby as much as your first child. Do not worry. When your new child is born, you will be adding love to love. You will discover a whole new source of unlimited love.

You may find yourself wondering, however, about how your first child will adjust to the new baby, and this concern will linger. Following are some helpful techniques passed along by women who have had two or more children.

Anticipating Jealousy

You should certainly expect to see some jealousy. It is normal and inevitable. As a matter of fact, you should be more concerned if your first child displays *no* jealousy. A first child will naturally feel somewhat displaced by the new baby. But here are some things you can do about it.

• Encourage him to verbalize his feelings so you will have the chance to offer reassurance.

• Offer your first child reassurance about your never-changing love for him. Assure him that you love him because of the special person he is and that nobody in the world could ever replace him.

• Put his jealous feelings into perspective by reminding him of the time when he was the baby and the center of attention.

• Get out his baby book and look it over with him in great detail. Share warm and detailed stories about his infancy. Show him pictures of himself as a baby, of you holding him

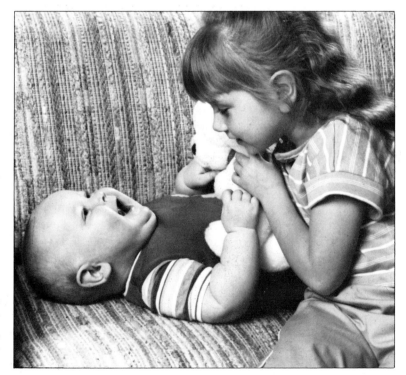

Reassure your first child about your never-changing love for her. Then watch her grow to love the newest member of the family.

97

and especially of you nursing him. It is wonderful to have at least one picture of you nursing each baby. It means a great deal to the toddler since he sees this as concrete evidence that you did for him what you are doing for the new baby.

• As you go about caring for your new baby and as your older child follows you, constantly tell him stories of his babyhood. As you change your new baby's diaper, say "I remember when I used to change your diapers. You used to play with a little rubber duck and chatter in baby talk as I changed you." As you rock your baby say, "I remember when I used to rock you like this; you used to reach up and hold my hair in your little hand." As you nurse your baby say, "You were such a good nurser when you were little. You used to drink my milk so fast. I knew you loved it and I loved nursing you."

All of this will help remind your older child of when you gave him the very same kind of care that he is so jealous of now. Helping him remember this allows him to feel secure about your love for him and to feel better about not being your baby any longer.

Accepting Regression

The natural excitement that accompanies the addition of a new baby to the family makes a clear statement to the older child: babies are highly valued, and being a baby brings much praise. So it is typical for a first child to regress a bit when the new baby arrives. Although this may occur right away, it could also appear when the new baby is about six months old, displays more personality and receives a great deal of attention for it.

This regression could take a number of forms. Many children who were previously potty trained may begin to wet their pants, cry more and have more temper tantrums. Bedtime may require extra patience and reassurance. Some toddlers even begin to talk in baby talk.

The most helpful way to handle this regression is to go along with it. Even refer to your "big" child as "my tiny baby" if he likes it. Reprimanding him for regressive behavior and telling him to act "like a big boy" will make him feel rejected and not solve the problem. Try to understand your child's babyish behavior and his reasons for doing so. It is never long lived.

Renewed Interest in Nursing

Most toddlers who are siblings of nursing babies will ask if they can nurse too. It is obvious even to a young child that nursing is more than giving food—the warmth and love that you give your baby are evident to the older child. They cannot help but want it too.

Go ahead and agree to let your toddler try to nurse. He will not remember how and he will not like the taste of warm breast-milk if he does get any, so the whole experiment will be over in a matter of seconds. What he really wants to know is if you are willing to include him in this wonderful love exchange. Knowing that instead of pushing him away, you were willing to include him, will satisfy him.

Who Comes First?

It may be difficult for your older child to adjust to the fact that the new baby's needs must come first. Since a newborn is completely helpless and has overwhelming needs, he cannot be asked to wait the way a two- or three-year-old can.

To solve the problem of an older child who demands attention, use a technique like the one we described earlier. When you need to go to the baby and when your older child feels resentful, tell him a story about a time when everything stopped because he cried. As you walk to your crying baby say, for example, "I remember when my friend was over and wanted me to visit with her but when you cried I said, 'Sorry, but my baby is crying and I have to go to him now.'"

Reminding him of the times you rushed to him while the world waited will help him to accept waiting for you while you attend to your new baby. And, of course, there will be some times when your toddler's needs are truly more pressing and he will come first.

Teaching Parenting

One of the real benefits of breastfeeding a new baby is that you can provide some parent education to the older child, who will absorb many valuable lessons quite naturally.

• Your child will learn that breastfeeding is the "normal" way to feed a baby. He will also sense that the breasts are a natural, healthy part of a woman's anatomy.

• Your older child will learn the importance of putting the baby's needs first and that a baby's cry is not to be ignored but responded to seriously. Do not be surprised if he asks you to rush over and nurse every crying baby he hears in the supermarket!

• Despite his feelings of jealousy, he will also learn to love the baby, and he will imitate the gentle nurturing he sees you give the baby. Many toddlers watch lovingly and gently stroke "their baby" as he nurses.

Making Special Time

While we have stressed how to help your older child adjust to your involvement with the new baby, we also must acknowledge the importance of his needs. It is only natural at this time for him to wonder if you still love him as much as you did before the new baby came. Sharing your love is not easy for him, but it will be easier if you can spend some time alone with him, as you did before the birth of the baby. You will be tired and you will face constant demands, so giving this extra attention to your older child will not be as easy as it sounds, but it is important and will pay off.

• Make a point of spending some focused time alone with your older child each day. Take advantage of your baby's nap or contented periods to give time to your toddler.

• If you are busy with the baby when your toddler demands your attention, ask him to wait, and promise to give him some time as soon as you are finished. Always follow through on this promise, and he will soon learn to trust and be satisfied with your offer.

• When your partner is home, ask him to care for the baby so that you and your toddler can play or even go on an errand together. Just talking to him and giving him your full attention for a short time will go a long way toward refueling his "emotional tank."

• Allow your older child to touch and handle the new baby. A certain amount of "germ exchange" is unavoidable and not harmful. The price you pay for overprotecting the new baby from your older child is greater in terms of resentment than the mild discomfort that results from the occasional cold that might be passed between the two children. Allowing your older child to help with the care of his sibling can be a source of pride for him. Let him bring you a diaper or apply some lotion to the baby's bottom. Of course, he will appreciate praise for his excellent help.

Preventing and Solving Breastfeeding Complications

Presenting the subject of breastfeeding difficulties is always a delicate task. On the one hand, reading about the wide range of possible breastfeeding complications may raise needless anxieties. On the other hand, your confidence in your ability to breastfeed may increase if you understand various possible complications—what causes them, how to prevent them and how to solve them. Knowing how to position your baby correctly, understanding the principle of supply-and-demand milk production, and having confidence in your ability to breastfeed is your best insurance against experiencing any difficulties.

The truth is, however, that most nursing women with some prior breastfeeding knowledge do not experience any serious complications. Just about any breastfeeding difficulty can be solved (and usually prevented). Only the rarest situation should actually interrupt or cause you to terminate your breastfeeding relationship. Please remember that our solutions are meant to help mothers and babies who are having these problems. Do not complicate your life by applying these measures to breast-feeding that is going well.

Engorgement

In the early days after your milk "comes in," you may feel a fullness and hardness in your breasts, called engorgement, that can be quite uncomfortable. This engorgement may be unpreventable and inevitable, especially with the first baby.

Causes • Extra milk in the breasts and extra blood in the tissue.

Prevention • Nurse early and often with no schedule and no time restrictions. You may be advised to limit your nursing schedule to prevent sore nipples. Sore nipples, however, are due to poor positioning of the baby at the breast, not to the amount of time she spends at the breast. (See pages 45 to 47.)

Solutions
• Hand-express a little milk before your baby latches on. (See how to on page 57.) Otherwise she will not be able to latch on well and nurse effectively.

• Keep your nursing unrestricted; you can offer the breast if you are uncomfortably full even if your baby is not demanding to be fed.

• Try warm compresses in between feedings for some comfort.

Plugged Duct

A plugged duct is a milk duct that has become obstructed. If you have a plugged duct, you will have a hard lump within your breast, which will feel inflamed and tender. A plugged duct can develop into a breast infection if it is not managed appropriately. For unknown reasons, some women simply seem more predisposed to plugged ducts. Caution: see your doctor if the lump does not disappear within a week.

Causes
• Insufficient emptying of the breasts.

• Restrictive clothing such as a tight bra, or wearing breast shields, especially during the night.

• The weather. Plugged ducts are more common in the winter, when cold air seems to make the muscle fibers in the areola and nipple contract, delaying the release of milk and leading to a blocked or plugged duct. Cold air also causes circulatory changes in the breasts and temperature changes in the glands, perhaps another contributing factor to a plugged duct.

Solutions
• Nurse often and long to empty your breasts better. Since you definitely want to empty the sore side, offer it first.

• Apply moist heat before a nursing. Even a hot shower is a good idea, since it will help your let-down reflex.

• During the nursing, gently massage your breast from the sore spot toward the nipple. You can also massage it during your hot shower, before putting your baby on the breast.

• Try changing positions when you nurse to help your baby more effectively reach all the milk ducts. Alternate between sitting up and lying down; even try the football hold (see page 48), especially if the plugged duct is located on the outer side of your breast.

• Try going braless if you can, or changing bra styles or sizes if you continue to have plugged ducts.

• Get some extra rest to allow your body's natural resources to fight against the possibility of a breast infection.

Breast Infection (Mastitis)

Like a plugged duct, a breast infection is a hard, inflamed, painful spot on your breast; additionally, however, you will have flu-like symptoms and a fever. Some women seem to have a predisposition to breast infections, for which there is no prevention. Caution: see your doctor if the lump does not disappear within a week.

Causes

• Stagnated milk that has been blocked in a duct or bacteria that has invaded the breast, perhaps through a cracked nipple.

Prevention

• Try to prevent a plugged duct.

• Relieve a plugged duct as soon as possible, before it has a chance to turn into an infection.

• Try to avoid fatigue by napping when your baby naps.

Solutions

• Call your medical professional, who may want to prescribe antibiotics. If so, it is imperative that you take them for the full course. Sometimes, instead of antibiotics, some doctors may suggest taking 1000 mg of vitamin C four times a day.

• Get enough rest and drink a lot of liquids.

• Apply heat between nursings. Or try nursing your baby while soaking in a hot bath.

• Massage the sore area gently during the feeding.

• Continue nursing on the infected breast, since keeping it as empty as possible is imperative. Your baby will not be harmed, since the milk itself is not usually "infected," and antibodies will have formed in your milk to protect your baby specifically from the bacteria causing your infection.

• Try to empty the infected side especially well. If you are very sore, start nursing on the well side to initiate the let-down reflex, then switch to the sore side right away and nurse longer there.

• If necessary, take analgesics for pain.

Special Circumstances

"Epidemic" breast infection. A rare type of breast infection is the kind referred to as "epidemic"—one that may have originated in the hospital nursery and was passed to the mother through a cracked nipple. In such a case, a large amount of bacteria may be present in the milk. If tests show that bacteria levels are too high, your baby can be temporarily taken off that breast. The affected breast must be emptied with a breast pump for a few days.

Breast abscess. Another rare variation is a breast abscess, an infection that has come to a head near the surface of the breast. If the abscess does not open by itself, it needs to be incised and drained. If the incision is on a part of the breast that would not come into contact with your baby's mouth, you can nurse on the infected side once the abscess drains. Otherwise, offer your baby only the unaffected side and pump the drained side for a few days.

Sore Nipples

A sore nipple usually feels like a burn on the surface of the nipple skin. Occasionally, the skin will also be cracked. A sore nipple usually lasts a few days, but can persist for a week or more. (Some women also use the term sore nipples to refer to pain inside the nipple at the beginning of the nursing.)

Prevention

• Make sure your baby is positioned properly at the breast. Incorrect positioning is by far the most prominent cause of sore nipples. (See the step-by-step guidelines on pages 46-47.)

• Alternate between sitting up and lying down to nurse. (See page 48.) If you find you prefer one position over another, wait until you are past the first few weeks before using it predominantly.

• After a nursing session, let any milk that is on your nipples dry in the air; the milk itself is good for the skin on your nipples.

• Apply a thin coat of hydrus lanolin or A and D ointment during the first two weeks to speed up healing, but be careful not to smother your nipples; they need air, too. (Some authorities do not feel the application of ointment is especially helpful.)

• Clean your nipples with water only; do not use soap or alcohol. The small protrusions on your areola, called Montgomery glands, secrete a natural cleansing substance that keeps your areola and nipples clean. Soap and alcohol wash away this protective fluid.

• Change nursing pads (and bra if necessary) whenever they are wet. Your nipples need to be dry. Do not use plastic-lined nursing pads, since they keep the moisture in and the healing air out.

• Make sure your areola is soft enough so your baby can get your nipple far back into her mouth. A very full breast may cause your baby to suck on the nipple alone, which is painful. Simply hand-express a little milk if your breasts are overfull before letting your baby latch on.

• After a nursing session, break the suction gently. (See page 46.)

• Do not use a bicycle-horn-type breast pump to express milk. This pump is generally ineffective and can cause sore nipples.

Solutions

Sore nipples are a common, although not very serious problem. Because they are so troublesome, we offer an extensive catalog of cures. All of them will not help you, but some will. Always remember the basic principles: position your baby correctly at the breast and keep your nipples dry. Also remember, sore nipples always go away!

Nursing Positions

• Correct your baby's position. Check all points of the positioning process. (See page 46.)

• Support your breast in your baby's mouth with your free hand. Even if you position your baby correctly at first, the weight of a heavy breast is more than a small baby can support with suction alone. An unsupported breast can slip out of its centered position during the feeding.

• Alternate positions from one feeding to the next. If changing between sitting and lying down is not enough, try the football hold. (See page 48.)

Dry Nipples

• Expose your nipples to air as much as possible, even to sunlight if you can. Be careful not to get sunburned, however.

• Try putting a wire tea strainer in your bra to keep air circulating around your nipples.

• Give your nipples a heat treatment: hold your hair dryer (on a low setting) about an arm's length away from your nipples and warm them gently a few times a day. Or, expose your nipples to a 60 watt bulb at a distance of 18 inches for 20 minutes four times a day.

Applying Preparations

• Nature's own preparation is fine. Rub those last drops of breast milk into your nipples; they have a healing effect.

• Apply a thin coat of hydrus lanolin or A and D ointment after air-drying your nipples. (However, if you are allergic to wool, do not use any products containing lanolin since it is extracted from sheep's wool and will irritate your skin. Also, don't use lanolin if you have a cracked nipple; lanolin softens the skin and seems to allow the crack to be pulled open more easily.)

• Try using unscented Chap Stick, vitamin E squeezed from a capsule, or gel from an aloe vera leaf. Apply it sparingly and wipe off the excess just before you nurse your baby. (Products that contain alcohol, perfumes or scents, or petroleum jelly, however, are not helpful and can make sore nipples worse.)

• Sponge your nipples with wet tea bags and then let them air-dry. Soak the tea bag in hot water (have a cup of tea!), then let it cool until it is comfortable on your skin. But remember that tea can stain bras and nightgowns.

Nursing Management

• When your nipples are sore, switch to short, frequent nursings.

• Try to anticipate your baby's hunger by nursing a little before she demands it. That way she will not approach your breast with a ravenous appetite and a strong suck.

• Offer the side that is least sore first.

• Hand-express a little milk before you nurse, so your baby will not have to suck so hard to initiate the let-down reflex.

• If you are unbearably sore, skip a feeding or two from the sore side. Hand express, instead, to prevent engorgement and maintain your milk supply. You may also need to offer your baby a pacifier to meet some of her sucking needs.

Pain Relief

• Use the breathing exercises you learned in your childbirth classes as your baby latches on. They will help you handle the pain and help you relax.

• Try relieving the discomfort with ice, since sore nipples resemble the pain you would experience with a burn. Ice treatments can be especially helpful just before a nursing.

• Try a pain-relief medication.

Flat Nipples

Nipples that protrude very little or not at all—flat nipples—can cause a new baby to have some problems latching on, since she may have trouble identifying the nipple if it does not protrude. Some babies, however, are not bothered at all by flat nipples. (See illustration in Chapter 2.)

Prevention

• None.

Solutions

• The hormones of pregnancy may extend flat nipples somewhat.

• Wear breast shields during the last three months of your

pregnancy. Breast shields exert an even and continuous pressure, which will gradually draw out your nipples. They are comfortable and inconspicuous to wear and can be purchased in some pharmacies and infant stores or ordered from La Leche League.

• Wear breast shields for ten minutes before each nursing.

• In the beginning, when your baby is learning to nurse, put ice on your nipple just before the feeding. Ice will make your nipple skin cold and more erect, and your baby will be able to find it more easily. Or, if you prefer, roll your nipple by hand to make the skin more erect. (You can give up this practice once your baby has learned how to latch onto the nipple.)

• If at all possible, avoid giving a bottle to your baby, especially during the early weeks. Because the contrast between the protruding rubber nipple and a mother's flat nipple is so pronounced, your baby may be especially prone to nipple confusion.

Inverted Nipples

Inverted nipples retract rather than protrude when the area behind the nipple is compressed, making it difficult for a baby to identify the nipple, latch onto it and draw it into the back of her mouth. (See illustration in Chapter 2.)

Prevention • None.

Solutions • During pregnancy, do what are called Hoffman's exercises to try to separate the adhesions that can sometimes cause inversion. To do these exercises, first imagine a plus sign on your nipple, then place your thumbs along the horizontal line at the base of your nipple. Press in with your thumbs and pull them away from each other. Then do the same along the

Hoffman's Exercises

Imagine a plus sign on your nipple. Place your thumbs along the horizontal line at the base of your nipple (left). Press in with your thumbs and pull them away from each other. Then do the same movement along the vertical line (right).

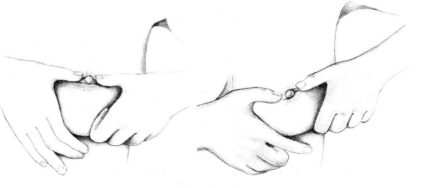

vertical line. Do this exercise about five times in each direction at least once a day during your pregnancy.

• Grasp your nipple and tug it forward to stretch the tiny muscles in the nipple.

• Wear breast shields during pregnancy. Start wearing them during your third month (or whenever you discover you have inverted nipples) for a few hours a day and increase the time up to eight hours a day; do not sleep in them, however. Give your nipples an occasional 20-minute air break when you are wearing shields. During the early days of nursing, you may still need to wear them between feedings until your baby is pulling your nipples out well.

• Try ice treatments, as you would if you had flat nipples. (See page 107.) Applying ice to your nipples just before you nurse will make them more erect, allowing your baby to latch on more easily.

Blister on Your Nipple

A blister may develop on your nipple, usually on the end.

Causes   • The nipple is probably not being properly centered in your baby's mouth.

Solutions   • Try to improve your nursing position, especially when you center the nipple before your baby latches on.

• Leave the blister alone; it is not serious and will heal itself.

• If you have any reason to suspect herpes, especially if you see a cluster of small blisters instead of just one, have a culture done to rule out herpes.

Thrush

Thrush is a type of yeast infection that is sometimes called Monilia. It thrives in warm areas such as the baby's mouth and the mother's breast, and it also thrives on milk. In your baby's mouth, thrush will look like a white-coated tongue and curds inside her cheeks, and she may have diaper rash, too. You will have persistently sore nipples and breast pain between feedings. Also, your nipples may be itchy, pink and flaky, and you may also have a vaginal yeast infection.

Causes   • Taking antibiotics, which may create an environment conducive to the growth of thrush.

• Taking oral contraceptives, which may also be a contributing factor.

• Catching it in the birth canal.

• Nursing someone else's baby, or letting babies share toys that go in the mouth.

Solutions

• Contact your doctor, who will probably prescribe an antibiotic ointment called Mycostatin Suspension. Be sure to treat both the baby's mouth and your breasts for the full two weeks.

• Try this home remedy, which will also clear up thrush. Treat thrush persistently in both mother and baby until it is completely gone.

For your baby's mouth: Dissolve one teaspoon of baking soda in one cup of water that is room temperature. Using clean cotton or a gauze pad, thoroughly wipe the inside of your baby's mouth, especially the tongue, inside the cheeks, and around the gums. Do this after every nursing. Make a fresh solution each day and stir it before each use.

For your nipples: Mix one tablespoon of vinegar with one cup of water and bathe your nipples in this solution after each nursing.

• While you are attempting to get rid of a thrush infection, pay special attention to cleanliness. Wash your hands well, and boil pacifiers and toys that go in your baby's mouth.

Faulty Let-Down Reflex

A faulty let-down reflex is when your milk production is normal but something interferes with the release of oxytocin and milk is not ejected or is only partially ejected through the duct system.

Causes

• Stress in the form of extreme shock, fright, worry or fatigue. Even then, the effect would be only temporary.

• Substances (when consumed in large amounts) like alcohol, nicotine or caffeine.

• A weak nurser.

Solutions

• Try to build up your confidence in your ability to breastfeed. Read and talk to breastfeeding friends; find support.

• Create as stress-free an environment for yourself as possible. Get comfortable, remove distractions (for instance, delay visits from upsetting or nonsupportive relatives). Put on your favorite music, do some breathing exercises and try to relax.

• Create a routine to help condition your let-down reflex. Every time you sit down to nurse do two other things before beginning, and follow the same pattern each time. For example, stretch your arms and shoulders, take a drink of water, then put your baby to the breast. Your let-down of milk should soon become conditioned to your pattern and will start sooner.

• When you feel a let-down of milk between nursings, put your baby to the breast so you become conditioned to this association.

• If you have an extreme let-down reflex problem, try nursing on a schedule as long as it is not harmful to your baby. To assist your conditioning, you may want to nurse every two or every three hours consistently until your reflex improves.

• If all else fails, your doctor can prescribe syntocinon, an artificial form of oxytocin, which stimulates the let-down reflex. It comes in a nasal spray and can be very effective for occasional use. However, prolonged use may render it ineffective, and it may eventually inhibit your natural let-down reflex.

Too Strong Let-down Reflex

If your let-down reflex is too strong, the force of your milk spray may cause your baby to gasp and sputter. As she grows older, however, she will be able to keep up with the force of the milk.

Prevention   • None.

Solutions   • When the let-down reflex occurs, take your baby off the breast for a minute and let the initial spurt of milk spray into a tissue or diaper. Then put your baby back on the breast. She may cough to clear her airway and then nurse eagerly again.

• To prevent your breasts from getting overfull, wake your baby for an occasional unscheduled feeding.

Low Milk Supply

If your let-down reflex is working but your baby is not gaining weight, seems dissatisfied and wets fewer than six to eight diapers a day, your problem may be a low milk supply.

Note, however, that genuine supply problems are quite rare. You should not mistake any of the following for a milk supply problem: a growth spurt, softer breasts, less leaking milk, a let-down reflex that feels less intense, a baby who is fussy but gains and produces wet diapers or a baby with an unusually strong sucking urge. In fact, these are normal parts of your continuing nursing relationship and do not indicate a supply problem.

If you have eliminated all of these possibilities and still feel that you have a low milk supply, consider whether any of the following might be the cause of your problem.

Causes

• Limited nursing—either restricted time at the breast or supplementation with bottles of formula or water. If the baby nurses less, you will produce less milk.

• Starting solids too soon, causing the baby to nurse less and your milk supply to drop.

• Taking birth control pills, which, in addition to passing hormones to your baby via your milk, will decrease your milk supply.

• Fatigue.

• A new pregnancy, which will reduce your milk, eventually replacing it with lower-volume colostrum.

• A low thyroid level.

• Substances found to or suspected of lowering milk supply: vitamin B_6, antihistamines, diuretics, heavy smoking and large amounts of caffeine.

• An extremely poor diet. Generally a poorly nourished woman can produce an adequate quantity and quality of milk; however, her protein intake can affect the volume of milk produced.

Solutions

• Nurse more often and for longer periods. Very frequent nursing should increase your milk supply within a couple of days.

• Offer both breasts at each nursing.

• Cut down on supplemental bottles or formula.

• Pump after the feeding to stimulate your supply if your baby is too small or too weak to empty your breasts well.

• Cut back on your extra activities. Rest, eat well and drink fluids. Take especially good care of yourself until your supply is up.

Too Much Milk

Occasionally a woman has so much milk that her baby cannot begin to exhaust her supply. Excessive leaking can be a problem for this woman.

Prevention • Do not overdo pumping.

Solutions • Nurse on one side only at each feeding, and alternate the side you offer.

The Slow-Weight-Gain Baby

A baby is considered to be gaining too slowly, according to medical criteria, if she fits the following description: her weight is below the third percentile, her growth in length and head circumference drops, and she falls below a specified amount on a weight chart. Slow weight-gain babies are generally shriveled-looking and irritable.

Causes • A health problem that should be checked by a physician to rule out a physical condition causing her to gain weight slowly.

• A health or lactation problem in the mother that can be addressed by a physician.

• A baby who may be sleeping through the night, getting fewer feedings, and probably gaining less weight.

• A baby who may be filling up on bottles of calorie-free water, which takes the place of nutritious breast milk and is not necessary for a breastfed baby.

• Improper breastfeeding technique.

Solutions • Give your baby more time at the breast. Many women have heard that a breastfed baby gets most of her milk in the first five to ten minutes and is only sucking after that. This may be true for a three-month-old baby with a terrific suck, but it may not be true for a small baby or for a weak nurser. Give your baby more time if she still seems hungry or eager to nurse.

• Try the "switch and burp technique" for the weak or lazy nurser. Nurse your baby briefly—maybe three minutes—then either sit her up or put her over your shoulder to burp her, which will make her more alert. Then put her on the other side for about three minutes, burp, switch again and so on. By offering each side often during each feeding, you are giving your milk enough time to drain down to the sinuses and be available for your baby, who will get more milk with each suck. This technique will also strengthen her suck. Once you feel your baby's sucking is stronger, and she is getting more milk and gaining well, you can go back to normal nursing. Also read about the non-nutritive suck on page 111.

• Make sure you are positioning your baby properly. If your nipple is not in the back of your baby's mouth and she is not pumping the sinuses, she will not get much milk.

• If your baby falls asleep after nursing for only a short time, burp her, try to awaken her gently and get her to take more milk. If she has swallowed air with the milk, she may feel temporarily full.

• If your baby nurses for a short time and then puts her fingers in her mouth, she may not be getting enough milk and is satisfying her sucking urge with her fingers. Take her fingers out of her mouth and put her back on the breast.

• If you have put your baby on solids, you may have started too early. Some babies gain less weight on solids, which are less useful nutritionally to an immature digestive system than the breast milk they are replacing. If you think this might be your problem, try cutting back on solids and nursing more.

• Try using the Lact-Aid Nurser Trainer®, which allows you to supplement your baby with either formula or stored breast milk and, at the same time, keep your baby nursing at the breast. This device consists of a plastic bag that hangs around your neck on a cord, with a very thin rubber tube going from the bag of milk to your nipple. When the baby sucks at the breast, she also receives milk from the bag. In addition to supplying extra nourishment, the Lact-Aid can also improve the strength and frequency of a baby's suck; since milk is flowing into the baby's mouth, she has no choice but to suck in order to swallow.

Special Circumstances An extremely rare cause of a slow-weight-gain baby is deprivation (of nurturing as well as nourishing) by the mother. These mothers need to seek professional counseling and support.

The Baby Refuses One Breast

Occasionally, a baby will consistently refuse to latch onto either the right or the left breast. If this happens, do not let yourself become engorged on the refused side. Hand-express or pump enough to keep your breast fairly soft. Eventually, your persistence will win out.

Prevention • None.

Solutions • Use the football hold (see page 48), which lets you switch breasts while allowing your baby to keep the same cheek on your breast—as if she were on her "favorite" side.

• Pick her up while she is asleep and put her on her least favorite side.

The Fussy or Reluctant Nurser

This baby will not settle down contentedly at the breast, but squirms, fusses and fights. She either resists latching on or repeatedly pulls off.

Prevention

• None.

Solutions

• Express a little milk onto your nipple to entice your baby to latch on.

• Try wrapping your baby snugly in a receiving blanket. This may help some babies settle down, but it may frustrate others.

• Stand and sway while nursing.

• See your pediatrician to make sure there is no physical cause.

• Put your baby over your shoulder, rub her and drop your shoulder; relax and breath deeply. Try again.

• Try rubbing the back of your baby's knees.

• Rub her palm if your baby will not open her mouth.

• Remove any clothes that may be causing extra stimulation on her face and head. Your baby may have an extremely strong rooting reflex and she may be receiving too much stimulation from your blouse on her face.

• If you are holding the back of your baby's head in your hand, rest it instead in the crook of your arm.

• Try to comfort and calm your baby before starting to nurse.

Nursing Strike

A baby who goes on a "nursing strike" is one who suddenly refuses to nurse for several days, an event that is often mistaken for weaning, even though weaning would almost certainly not occur suddenly or when a baby is less than a year old. Although your baby will show clear disdain for nursing during this period, once the strike is over, she will nurse again with pleasure. Give your baby a great deal of cuddling and stroking during the nursing strike.

Causes

• Unknown. Some possibilities, however, are teething, a cold, a sore throat or an ear infection.

Solutions

• Pick up your baby when she is asleep and put her to the breast; most babies will automatically latch on. This may not work the first time, but keep trying; it will work eventually.

- Try nursing while walking.

- Cut back on solids and juices temporarily if your baby is less than a year old and on solids.

The Sleepy or Placid Baby

A nondemanding, easy-going, "good" baby may sleep for long periods and not gain weight well.

Causes
- A premature or very small baby.

- A mother who has been taking sedatives or consuming large amounts of alcohol.

- No cause. Usually this is just a baby's nature; as she grows older, she will be more alert.

Solutions
- Offer the breast at least every three hours (maybe every four during the night). Do not wait for your baby to demand.

- Take off your baby's clothes, except for her diaper, for the nursing. This increased skin-to-skin contact stimulates her and keeps her more awake. Touch and stroke your baby.

- Go to this type of baby as soon as she begins to fuss. You want to teach her that she can ask for her needs to be met and that you will respond to them.

- Squeeze some milk into your baby's mouth from your breast to get her started.

- Rub the back of her neck in a circular motion or rub down her spine to wake her. Or try stroking her toes or rubbing down her foot from her toes to her heel.

- Jiggle her if she seems to doze at the breast.

- Tug at your breast, if she stops sucking, to inspire some renewed sucking.

- Talk or sing to your baby; try to interact with her to stimulate her and keep her awake.

Biting

Babies occasionally bite either while they are nursing or when they let go of the breast. Contrary to popular belief, this is not a very common problem, regardless of the age of your baby or the number of teeth she has.

Causes
- The baby who is teething and has a tingling feeling in her gums after she creates suction.

• The baby who has fallen asleep and slipped off the nipple; she bites in an attempt to get back on.

Solutions • With your finger, press firmly along your baby's gums before putting her on your breast. This may eliminate the tingling feeling that could be causing her to bite.

• If your baby bites, say "ouch" or "no" with surprise. This may startle your baby enough to discourage her from doing it again.

• Your baby cannot bite while sucking because her tongue covers her bottom teeth. Toward the end of the feeding, watch for your baby's tongue to slide in. This may mean she will bite, so take her off the breast at that point.

• If your baby is asleep and you feel her sliding off, slip your finger in between her gums and your breast. She will bite your finger rather than your breast as she attempts to get back on.

Colicky Baby

A colicky baby will cry as if in pain for no apparent reason. She often cries at the same time every evening and usually pulls her legs up as she screams. No one knows for sure what colic is. It is probably one label for several problems, but it seems to disappear by itself by three months of age.

Causes • Gas pain or a digestive problem.

• The result of something the mother has eaten, like cabbage, milk or excess sugar.

• The result (in one view) of an immature digestive system or (in another view) of a too-mature digestive system.

• A result of no food intake by the mother between lunch and suppertime, and thus a lower milk volume in the evening.

• An overactive nervous system.

Solutions • Do not assume your baby has colic until your health-care provider has ruled out the possibility of a more serious health problem. Read *Crying Baby, Sleepless Nights*, by Sandy Jones, for more ideas along these lines.

• Hold, rock, walk and offer comfort to your baby during her distress. You cannot always quiet her, but it is important not to abandon her at this time.

• Try the "colic hold," which is soothing to many shrieking babies. Hold your baby across your forearm, with her stomach against your arm and her head near your hand. The firm

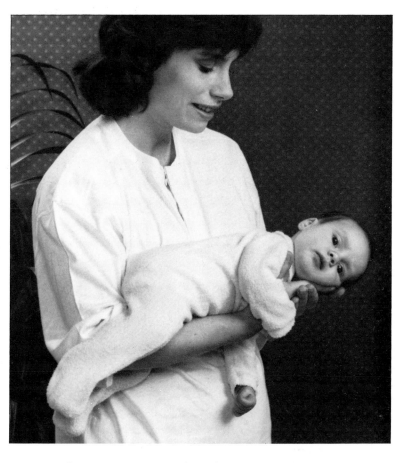

Colic Hold

Soothes many crying babies. Hold your baby across your forearm with her stomach against your arm and her head near your hand. The firm support of your arm against her abdomen is comforting.

support of your arm against her abdomen is comforting.

• Take your baby for a stroller ride or an ever-effective "snooze-cruise." Colicky babies are often soothed by motion.

• Turn on your vacuum—apparently its sound resembles intrauterine noises and will often quiet a crying baby. To make it almost foolproof, put your baby in a frontpack and actually vacuum. The combination of the closeness, the rocking motion and the sound will generally calm even the most hysterical baby.

• Place your baby in an infant seat on top of a running clothes dryer. The noise, vibration and gentle heat often quiet a colicky baby. Stay close by, however, to see that the vibrations do not cause the seat to slide off.

• Temporarily eliminate any vitamins that contain iron to see if it helps. Iron supplements in vitamins have been implicated in babies with digestive pain.

• Eliminate dairy products from your diet to see if your baby's condition improves. Many babies will react negatively to cow's milk products that are consumed by the mother and passed through her milk.

• Eliminate or cut down your intake of caffeine and nicotine.

• Watch what you drink. Carbonated beverages consumed by the mother can cause gas in some babies; herbal teas cause problems for others. Also, grain beverages may produce gas.

• If your baby has a gas problem, think about foods you may be eating that give you gas. Consider broccoli, cabbage, turnips, cauliflower, beans, sugar or chocolate. Even an excess of fresh fruits like melon and peaches can cause gas in some mothers and babies.

• Try burping your baby more. Some babies take in air while nursing, which causes them discomfort later. If your baby gulps loudly during the let-down of milk, she is probably taking in air. Take her off the breast during the "big rush" at let-down, then put her back on.

• If your colicky baby is crying and will not accept the breast as comfort, offer a pacifier in addition to holding or rocking her.

• Your pediatrician may prescribe medication for your colicky baby.

Jaundice

Jaundice is a condition caused by the accumulation of bilirubin in the newborn's blood. Its primary symptom is a yellowing of the baby's skin, eyes, mucous membranes and excretions. Jaundice is not a disease itself, but a symptom of immature liver function. The bilirubin that is present in the newborn's blood is a by-product of the breakdown of the old blood cells that a baby is normally born with. Blood cells that break down are usually eliminated by the liver, but for a variety of possible reasons, a newborn's liver may not be able to handle these demands.

Jaundice is a common condition in newborns, and it goes away with time. There is no evidence that bilirubin levels lower than 20 mg/dl during the first three days after birth and lower than 25 mg/dl after the third day have any harmful effect on a full-term healthy infant.

There are three basic categories of neonatal jaundice.

• Normal **physiologic jaundice,** the most common type, affects perhaps half of all newborn infants (whether they are breast or bottlefed); it appears on the second to fourth day after birth. Normal physiologic jaundice results from the rapid breakdown of excess fetal red blood cells and the inability of the liver to excrete the excess ineffectively in the first few days of life.

• **Pathologic jaundice** is abnormal and may be caused by several conditions, among which are Rh or ABO blood incompatibilities. Pathologic jaundice, which is visible at birth or within the first 24 hours, is quite rare.

• **Breast milk jaundice,** which is also extremely rare, is thought to be caused by an unidentified factor in the milk of a very few women. If your baby is breastfed, a case of normal physiologic jaundice may sometimes mistakenly be called breast milk jaundice. But there are crucial differences between the two: breast milk jaundice does not become visible until the fifth through seventh days after birth or even the second week of life. It can last from up to three to ten weeks.

Causes

Many factors can affect a newborn's ability to clear bilirubin.

• The amount of plasma proteins in the baby's bloodstream that are available to pick up and bind the bilirubin for conjugation and excretion. These plasma proteins are produced in the liver from the nutrients in breast milk.

• The maturity of the baby's liver, which affects its ability to conjugate bilirubin. The mother's nutrition during her pregnancy will partially determine the functioning level of her baby's liver after birth.

• The presence of certain medications in the mother. Medications that the mother received during labor pass into the baby's system and must be eliminated. Some medications (valium, oxytocin and epidural anesthesia have been implicated) compete with bilirubin for binding sites on the plasma proteins or for conjugation by liver enzymes.

• Supplementation of a breastfed baby with water or glucose water. Breast milk is high in the specific proteins required for good liver function, but they are not present in water or glucose water, which are sometimes given to a jaundiced newborn. While some health professionals think that water will "flush" the jaundice out of a baby's system, providing water instead of protein actually contributes to, rather than solves, the problem of jaundice.

• An infection in the baby that introduces bacteria that may compete with bilirubin for detoxification by the liver. Again this slows down the elimination of bilirubin and thus prolongs the jaundice.

• Intravenous fluids received by the mother during labor and delivery. These fluids, which pass through the placenta into the baby's blood, can dilute the electrolytes in the infant's blood; the red blood cells then absorb extra water, swell, and can burst, releasing the cell's hemoglobin and raising the bilirubin count higher.

• Bruises on the baby, which introduce an extra number of destroyed blood cells into her system, require more work by her liver, and interfere with the elimination of the bilirubin.

Solutions • Continue to nurse your baby frequently. Breastfeeding does not need to be discontinued in any jaundiced, healthy, full-term infant. Studies have shown that babies who nurse at least every three hours or more often have lower serum bilirubin levels than those babies who nurse less often. Frequent nursings will also encourage the rapid passing of a baby's stool and thus prevent the reabsorption of this bilirubin from the meconium (or early stool). Also, do not supplement your breast milk with water or formula. Research has demonstrated that supplements do not lower the bilirubin levels of breastfed infants.

• If your baby has a severe case of jaundice, your doctor may place her under fluorescent lights sometimes referred to as "bililights," which seem to speed up the elimination of bilirubin. This procedure is probably overused for cases of normal jaundice, where the level of bilirubin is not dangerous.

• Try home remedies, which include undressing your infant and exposing her to daylight from a window (but not direct sunlight, which can cause sunburn), or placing a new fluorescent daylight tube that is about sixteen inches long over her crib.

• Some authorities will want to temporarily (for 12 to 24 hours) discontinue breastfeeding only in the rare cases of breast milk jaundice. For those missed nursings, the baby can be fed breast milk from another mother. It is never necessary to terminate breastfeeding permanently because of jaundice.

Summary

We have attempted to include the difficulties that have any likelihood of developing. Again, let us stress that you will probably experience no breastfeeding difficulties at all. If you should experience a problem and need more help than we have provided here, call your health-care provider if he or she is knowledgable about and supportive of breastfeeding. Also, call your local La Leche League Leader, who will have tremendous resources available to help you.

Chapter Eight Special Situations

Occasionally a mother faces a special circumstance that requires her to change the management of her breast-feeding. Happily, situations like this are rare, but their implications for the health of mother and baby are often rather complicated. In this chapter, we will present and discuss a few of these special situations. Our discussion, however, is intended only to supply information and not to take the place of proper medical guidance. Always seek appropriate medical care when it is necessary. And if you need support in any situation, seek it out. La Leche League can often put you in touch with other mothers who have experienced a similar problem.

If Your Baby Is Premature

There are basically two kinds of small babies and their special needs are somewhat similar. A premature baby (often called a preemie, for short) is one born prior to 37 weeks of gestation; his weight and length are normal for his gestational age. A low-birth-weight baby—called Small for Gestational Age (SGA)—is one born closer to term or at term; his weight and length are below normal limits for his gestational age. We will discuss some basic principles for all low-birth-weight babies; your medical professional can advise you about your particular situation.

How It Affects Nursing

• These babies need all their energy for growth and are often too weak to suck.

• They tend to have more fragile digestive tracts, and they are more prone to infection, especially of the respiratory tract.

• They have special nutritional needs: more protein for growth, and more sodium, chloride and calcium.

• The mother is usually fine, and her milk supply is not affected.

• Very small babies are usually fed by a tube to their stomachs. A somewhat larger baby can usually be bottlefed with a special nipple. Generally, babies over five-and-a-half pounds can begin to nurse at the breast, but are often weak and slow to learn.

What Can Be Done
Before Your Baby Can Nurse

• If you plan to breastfeed your premature or small baby, you should begin pumping soon after birth, so that your baby can receive your colostrum and your milk, either by tube or bottle. As the mother of a premature baby, your milk differs from that of a mother who delivers at term. It is higher in many of the nutrients that a preemie needs, so it is better for a preemie than milk from a donor or from a milk bank pool. However, a preemie may still need supplements of such nutrients as iron, folic acid, vitamin D, calcium or vitamin C.

• When pumping milk for your preemie, you can expect ups and downs in your supply. You will need to relax as much as possible and accept all the support and encouragement you can get from your family and the hospital staff.

• Even before your baby can nurse, you should be allowed and encouraged to have as much physical contact with him as possible. It is good for the baby and greatly aids the bonding process, which may be slower with a preemie, due to his condition and the separation that is often necessary.

Once You Begin To Nurse

You may begin to nurse your baby while he is still in the hospital, but breastfeeding will really become established once you bring him home.

• Once your baby can begin to nurse, you enter an important transition period. He will still be weak and inefficient at the breast, and he may be recovering from an illness. Both of you will be learning how to nurse and probably adjusting to living at home without the guidance of hospital staff.

• The weight and size of your baby need not be the only factors that determine when he is ready to go home. Encourage your medical professional to consider other important clues like these: Are his vital signs stable? Does he have any significant health abnormalities? Is his feeding going well (either by bottle or at the breast)? Are you healthy? Are you and your partner informed and prepared to take care of him?

• Your patience, understanding and perseverance will help you learn how to best meet your tiny baby's needs. You may supplement with bottles of breast milk for a period while your supply regulates and your baby gains strength enough to nurse on his own. If you need to, try stimulating a let-down reflex before he nurses so that he receives milk as soon as he sucks. If he is sleepy at the breast, try to stimulate him a bit with skin-to-skin contact or gentle prodding, like rubbing the soles of his feet.

It is easy to concentrate on your baby's problems when he has special needs. Try instead to focus on his health and normalcy. Despite a difficult and slow start, he soon will be a happy, healthy child.

If Your Baby Has a Cleft Lip or Palate

The word cleft means "opening or split." A cleft can occur in a baby's upper lip, the hard palate (or roof) near the front of the mouth, the soft palate nearer the back of the mouth, or in a combination of the lip and palate. About one-quarter of all clefts are in the lip, one quarter are in the palate, and about half involve the lip and palate together.

How It Affects Nursing

• A baby with a cleft lip or palate has a diminished ability to latch on and suck well at the breast. Suction can occur only with a tight seal, which is difficult when there's an opening. A cleft in the soft palate may be undetected until you notice that your baby does not seem to be nursing well. Your first clue may be that he does not seem to be able to create enough suction to keep the nipple in his mouth.

• Some babies with clefts, on the other hand, nurse quite well, and a bottle may be more difficult because the flow is too fast.

• Often when a baby with a cleft nurses, milk runs into his nasal passage and out of his nose. Babies usually do not seem to mind this and it poses no real problem.

• Babies with clefts are often prone to respiratory infections, making the health benefits of breast milk of particular importance.

What Can Be Done

Mothers of cleft babies are always far better at feeding them than hospital personnel are. At first it may feel tedious and awkward to nurse a baby with a cleft. But you will quickly learn how to feed your own baby effectively, and it will feel easy and comfortable. Remember, your baby is normal; he just needs reconstructive surgery, which will usually be performed when the baby is six to fourteen months old, depending on his health and the extent of the cleft. This may be an especially difficult time. (See the section on the hospitalized baby, pages 127 and 128.)

• Some babies nurse well when pressure is applied from the breast against the cleft to fill the gap and help create better suction.

• Incline your baby's head a bit so the milk will run easily down his throat and not into the nasal cavity, or use the French position (see illustration), which makes it very easy for these babies to swallow.

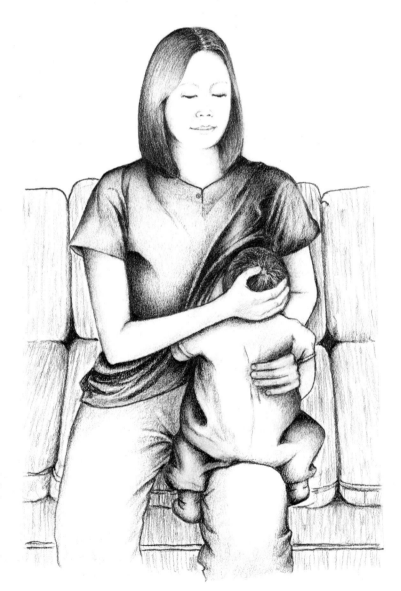

French Position

At first it may feel awkward to nurse a baby with a cleft. Place your baby on your knee facing your breast. The French position makes it easier for these babies to swallow. Soon it will feel easy and comfortable.

• If your baby nurses better on one side than the other, try using the football hold on the other side. (See page 48.)

• If your baby seems to be able to nurse well but has trouble maintaining enough suction to keep the nipple in his mouth, you may need to actually hold the breast to his mouth, just as you would a bottle.

If Your Baby Is Mentally Handicapped

Your physician may diagnose a mental handicap at birth or the signs of this handicap may gradually reveal themselves, allowing later detection. Whether the handicap is slight or severe, it could have an effect on your baby's ability to nurse. It should not, however, make breastfeeding impossible. Nursing will help you accept and fall in love with your baby. Providing the nurturing and nourishment only you can give will help you feel better about yourself and your child.

How It Affects Nursing

• Your baby may be slow to react to stimuli and slow to learn, even to nurse.

• Your baby's reflexes may be affected, including the sucking reflex, which is necessary for breastfeeding. This may mean a difficult start, but he can learn to nurse, given your patience and perseverance.

• Some mentally handicapped babies (for instance, those with Down's Syndrome) are more prone to respiratory infections, making breastfeeding especially valuable.

• Other complications—like a small mouth or a thick or retracting tongue—may hamper a baby's ability to nurse.

• The bonding process is often affected, and some mothers reject the baby initially. Mothers begin to fall in love with a fantasy of their baby during pregnancy, and often find it hard to let themselves fall in love with a baby who is less perfect than the fantasy. Often, too, they fear the loss of the baby due to a medical problem or to an institution, so they hold back their natural love for the child.

What Can Be Done

• By all means, breastfeed your baby, and seek out support and guidance for the concerns of your baby, yourself and your family. In many ways, you will be called upon to exhibit great patience and understanding.

• Remember that the perfect nutrition of breast milk will help your baby develop to his maximum potential. And the extended skin contact associated with nursing is the wonderful stimulation your baby needs.

If Your Baby Has Diarrhea

Diarrhea is an intestinal disorder characterized by extremely loose, often foul-smelling, bowel movements. This is a rare condition in a totally breastfed baby, so do not mistake your baby's normal yellow (sometimes greenish), watery stools for diarrhea. True diarrhea will usually smell foul and often contain mucus. In a breastfed baby it will often be almost pure liquid, without the curds you see in a normal stool.

How It Affects Nursing

•Nursing can continue without interruption. You may be told to temporarily discontinue breastfeeding, but this is not necessary unless your baby cannot take anything, even water, by mouth.

• Your baby may be fussy at the breast and want to nurse less (or more), depending on his specific condition and other symptoms. If your baby is severely dehydrated, consult your physician.

• A baby with diarrhea will pass off a lot of fluid and may dehydrate easily. The best clues to dehydration are skin that is dry to the touch and a lethargic baby.

What Can Be Done

• Nurse as often and as long as you can. Breast milk's high water content will help replace fluid lost with diarrhea. Breast milk also provides perfect nutrition, which is what your baby needs to recover as quickly as possible.

• If your medical professional advises you to stop nursing and start feeding water with flavored gelatin or Pedialyte, ask about continuing breast milk instead. A baby who can take anything by mouth, even water, can take breast milk.

• Sometimes a bit of water by mouth or some small ice chips can help a baby feel better and help prevent dehydration.

• Some health professionals recommend an enema for dehydration since it is a faster way to get fluid into a baby than by offering water or breast milk by mouth. For a very dehydrated baby, this may be an effective solution.

If Your Baby Has a Fever

A fever, or an elevated body temperature, is a sign that the body is fighting an infection. Because the intensity of the fever does not necessarily correspond to the severity of the infection, a baby may have a high fever with a very minor illness or a low fever with a rather serious condition. Since a fever is the body's way of fighting infection, it is not always necessary (and sometimes inappropriate) to control a fever.

How It Affects Nursing

• A fever may make your baby uncomfortable and that may change his nursing pattern. He may be too miserable to nurse, or he may nurse much more for comfort.

• Dehydration can be a problem, so see that your baby gets plenty of fluids, preferably breast milk.

What Can Be Done

• Continue breastfeeding, if at all possible. If your baby can have anything by mouth, even water, he can have breast milk. This is his best source of nourishment for recovery and his best source of comfort as well.

• Up to 102 degrees Fahrenheit (rectally), let a fever do its work and do not try to control it. Help your baby feel comfortable with light clothing and a cool room.

• A fever of 102 to 104 degrees (F.) is still not too dangerous, but it may make your baby more uncomfortable. A cool, wet washcloth makes a good compress for his face and chest, and it is usually all that is necessary to manage the fever and help your baby feel better.

• When a fever reaches 104 degrees (F.) or above it is necessary to seek medical advice about medication to control it. You may be advised to administer liquid acetaminophen orally or by rectal suppository if your baby is vomiting. A fever becomes dangerous to your baby's health when it reaches 106 degrees (F.).

• Lethargy and a very dry skin are signs of dehydration, which is possible when a baby has a fever. Usually this will be prevented if you are nursing a lot and offering occasional sips of water and ice chips.

If Your Baby Is Hospitalized

Your baby may require hospitalization, either immediately after birth or at some later point. Breastfeeding is a source of comfort to both mother and baby during this difficult and stressful time. The effect on breastfeeding is determined to a great degree by the condition that made hospitalization necessary.

How It Affects Nursing

• In most cases, hospitalization will mean limited nursing or no nursing for a period of time. If this is the case, you can resume nursing as soon as your baby is better.

• While a sick baby will often have less desire to nurse (although some want to nurse much more), he should be held, rocked and cuddled for comfort if possible.

• Because of the possibly erratic breastfeeding schedule, your milk supply may be low.

• Expect to be emotionally drained and physically fatigued, but remember this is only temporary.

What Can Be Done

• Nurse whenever possible—it is the best nutrition your baby can get. If you must stop nursing for a time, pump your breasts to keep up your supply, and maybe your baby can receive the milk you pump by tube or bottle.

• More than ever, this is a time when breastfeeding provides far more than nutrition. Nursing will help comfort you and your baby, and bring some sense of normalcy to a hectic, troubled time.

• Discuss the breastfeeding issue with your medical professional and the hospital staff. Let them know that continuing breastfeeding is very important to you, that you want to resume nursing as soon as possible, that you want to hold and cuddle your baby as much as you can, that you want your baby to receive breast milk for nourishment and that you want to avoid bottles if possible.

• If you can arrange it, stay with your baby around the clock. Some hospitals have arrangements for this; others may let you bring in a cot.

• Take care of yourself, too. Your sick baby needs a mother who is as rested and healthy as possible. When trying to stay calm, remember that this is only a temporary condition.

If You Have Diabetes

A diabetic is a person whose body does not properly produce insulin, which regulates blood sugar levels. Some diabetics can regulate blood sugar with only careful attention to diet, and some have to administer regular injections of insulin.

How It Affects Nursing

• Maternal diabetes need not change your decision to breastfeed, although the condition itself or the medication you take to control it may inhibit your let-down reflex to a degree.

• Because there may be wide fluctuations in your blood sugar, you may wonder if there is enough sugar in your milk. Be assured that your milk lactose level remains constant, in spite of variations in your blood glucose level.

• Your baby's changing demands for breast milk may change your blood sugar level, since milk production burns calories. However, most diabetic mothers find that their condition stabilizes and their need for insulin decreases during lactation.

• Breastfed babies are far less likely to be obese adults than are bottlefed babies. Since obesity can predispose a person to diabetes, this is a fact of particular importance to a diabetic mother who wants to reduce her baby's chances of developing the same condition.

What Can Be Done • Breastfeeding is clearly a very good choice for the diabetic mother. You will delight in breastfeeding, and you will feel like a "normal" mother after a high-risk pregnancy.

• Monitor your condition carefully during breastfeeding, especially the first week.

• More than ever, keep your meals regular, and eat frequent snacks. Prepare as many meals as you can refrigerate or freeze before your baby is born, to make regular meals easy after the baby has arrived.

• Enjoy the fact that your condition will probably be more stable while you are breastfeeding.

If You Have Had Breast Surgery

There are four types of breast surgery.

• **Silicone Augmentation**—the surgical placement in the breast of enclosed implants of silicone for cosmetic reasons. Injections of free-flowing silicone are now illegal in the U.S.

• **Reduction Surgery**—surgery performed to decrease breast size by the removal of breast tissue; such surgery may significantly reduce the size of the duct system.

• **Mastectomy**—the surgical removal of an entire breast, or both breasts, usually due to the presence of a cancerous growth.

• **Biopsy**—the surgical removal of a small portion of breast tissue, when malignancy is suspected, for examination and diagnosis.

How It Affects Nursing • **Silicone Augmentation.** A mother's ability to breastfeed is usually not impaired with silicone implants, although there are some complications that may interfere with the proper functioning of the breast. If ducts have been cut, you will produce less milk. If nerves have been cut, the resulting loss of sensation may impair let-down of milk. Silicone injections have also been known to cause scar tissue to develop around the duct system, often impairing the breasts' ability to lactate properly.

• **Reduction Surgery.** Provided the surgery was done carefully, reduction surgery should have only a limited effect on breastfeeding. As long as the nipple was not displaced and reattached, and enough of the secretory tissue and duct system remain, normal breastfeeding can take place.

• **Mastectomy.** If one breast remains, it can easily produce enough milk to breastfeed your baby.

• **Biopsy.** If the nipple was not cut, you need not wean. After a healing period, your baby will be able to nurse at the affected breast again.

What Can Be Done

• **Silicone Augmentation.** If you have had silicone implants, prepare for a normal breastfeeding experience. If you have had injections, you may or may not have difficulties from scar tissue. You may have a limited milk supply, which you can supplement with bottles or a Lact-Aid®.

• **Reduction Surgery.** If you have had reduction surgery, you can certainly try breastfeeding. You will soon know whether or not there has been damage that will keep you from continuing.

• **Mastectomy.** If you have had one breast removed, simply nursing at the other breast will cause it to produce plenty of milk for your baby.

• **Biopsy.** If you should require a biopsy, nurse again as soon as possible, usually just a few days after surgery. There will be some pain, but also physical relief at being able to empty the breast thoroughly. It may take some time to build up your supply again in that breast.

If You Have Accessory Nipples

A woman's breasts develop along a line of tissue called the "milk line," which runs from shoulder to groin. Sometimes an extra nipple—called an accessory nipple—develops, with or without breast tissue, along that line, most commonly near the underarm. This condition, known as hypermastia, is present in two to six percent of all women.

How It Affects Nursing

• Depending on the amount of secretory tissue present, an accessory nipple may or may not swell when your milk comes in, and there may or may not be some pain with this initial swelling. The nipple may even secrete drops of milk.

• Breastfeeding will not be affected in any way.

What Can Be Done

• If you experience no symptoms or difficulty with an accessory nipple, no special attention is required.

• If you do experience swelling or pain when your milk comes in, apply ice to reduce the swelling and relieve the pain. It may also help to apply compression with an elastic bandage. The swelling and discomfort will diminish and go away within a few days, and the nipple will return to its normal, prepregnancy state.

• Do not express milk from an accessory nipple, since doing so would cause nature's supply-and-demand system to produce more milk in that tissue, compounding the problem.

If You Are Ill

There are four general categories of illness that will have an effect on your ability to breastfeed.

• **Minor illnesses,** such as colds, flu and breast infections, that occur in a breastfeeding mother just as they would at any other time.

• **Serious illnesses,** such as pneumonia or mononucleosis.

• **Contagious conditions,** such as chicken pox, tuberculosis or herpes.

• **Hospitalization of the breastfeeding mother** due to illness or injury.

How It Affects Nursing

• **Minor Illness.** A minor illness may reduce your milk supply for a while, but plentiful nursing will bring it up again. You may be prone to dehydration, and you may feel it is difficult to get adequate rest for recovery while breastfeeding.

• **Serious Illness.** If you have a serious illness, your supply will probably be low and you will need plenty of rest, but breastfeeding can usually continue.

• **Contagious Condition.** If you have a contagious disease, your baby has already been exposed, so there is no point in separation. In the rare cases where the mother and baby must be separated, breastfeeding can often resume when the mother is no longer contagious.

• **Hospitalization of the Mother.** If you are hospitalized, the stress will undoubtedly affect your milk supply. Depending on the condition that required hospitalization, you may be temporarily separated from your baby.

What Can Be Done

• **Minor Illness.** Breastfeeding your baby while you rest and recover is easier if you and your baby go to bed together and nurse and sleep intermittently. Drink plenty of fluids to aid your recovery, prevent dehydration and boost your milk supply. Gradually resume your normal activity level after you are fully recovered.

• **Serious Illness.** This is an important time to get help for your family; you cannot recover while you are trying to cook and clean. With your baby in bed with you, you can both nurse and sleep around the clock. If you work outside the home, take as much time off as possible, so that you are fully recovered before you return.

• **Contagious Condition.** Special cautions about hygiene may be in order, depending on how your disease is transmitted. Your milk will offer your baby specific antibodies, so it is highly advantageous for nursing to continue. If nursing has to be interrupted, a good diet, lots of fluids and plenty of nursing will be important when it is resumed.

• **Hospitalization of the Mother.** If it is at all possible, delay going to the hospital until your baby is older. If hospitalization is imperative, arrange for your baby to stay at the hospital with you or to be brought to you for nursing several times a day. If breastfeeding is interrupted, use a breast pump temporarily and resume breastfeeding as soon as possible. Attention to diet and rest are essential.

General Principles

A breastfeeding mother who is ill never has an easy time of it, but there are some general principles that lead to a faster, more complete recovery and can help maintain breastfeeding.

• Since stress and fatigue are two crucial factors to contend with, do whatever it takes to allow yourself a peaceful recovery time.

• Nurse your baby, since you will probably find it a comfort, rather than a drain.

• Pay special attention to your diet and fluid intake, which aid your recovery and keep up your milk supply.

• If you are taking any medication, consult your medical professional, your pharmacist, or La Leche League about its safety during lactation. If you are advised to wean your baby, even temporarily, look for an alternate drug that will allow you to continue nursing.

• Weaning is rarely necessary, unless the illness is such a severe strain on the mother that she simply cannot handle it.

If You Become Pregnant

Although lactation generally suppresses ovulation, making it act as a natural birth control device, it is still possible to become pregnant while nursing. While this usually occurs when the first baby is older, eating solids, sleeping through the night and nursing less often, it can happen when he is still young and nursing around the clock.

How It Affects Nursing

• There are no statistics to show that breastfeeding during pregnancy is unhealthy. Unless you feel strongly about it, there is seldom reason to wean your baby if you become pregnant.

• During the course of your pregnancy, your milk supply will diminish and be replaced by colostrum.

• A common complaint of a pregnant nursing mother is a mysterious condition called the "empty breast sensation"—an odd mix of physical and emotional feelings. It is an uncomfortable but not painful sensation that is felt only when the baby is at the breast. Most mothers describe it as an incredible sense of urgency, although they cannot identify what they feel urgent about. The current medical explanation is that it is possibly caused by the partial collapse of ducts due to continued nursing with a decreasing milk supply. It usually occurs in the fifth month of pregnancy and may last several weeks or months.

• Suckling at the breast stimulates uterine contractions and may cause the onset of a premature labor if you are predisposed to it. If you are, it may be wise for you to wean.

• Another pregnancy clearly places a double stress on your body, especially if your first baby is very young and dependent on you for all his nutritional needs. (Your body is still recuperating from your last pregnancy and birth for as long as three years.)

• Sore nipples, which are common in pregnancy, can be particularly uncomfortable if you have a nursing baby.

• Pressure from outsiders is often negative and plentiful. To many, the sight of a pregnant woman nursing a baby is more than they can tolerate.

• Finding clothing that covers a pregnant tummy yet allows for discreet nursing requires great ingenuity!

What Can Be Done

• Some mothers choose to wean at some point in the pregnancy because they simply do not feel comfortable about the situation.

• Some babies, particularly older ones, wean themselves naturally as the milk supply diminishes. If this occurs late in pregnancy and if the mother allows it, some of these babies will resume nursing when the new baby is born and the milk supply increases. This poses no problems and the supply will pick up to meet the demands of both babies. Other babies continue nursing throughout the pregnancy and continue to nurse after the new baby arrives. (See Tandem Nursing, page

• Try the usual remedies to relieve sore nipples. They may work in this situation. (See page 104.) An older baby often will accept limited nursing when he understands that "mommy is too sore to nurse more right now."

• If you are being pressured to wean, but want to continue nursing, try to plan as much privacy for nursing as you can arrange. Breastfeeding is a private right that belongs to you and your baby, and you need not allow the attitudes of others to interfere. Often an older baby will accept that nursing is a "secret" and can wait to nurse until you have a few private moments.

• There seems to be no remedy for the "empty breast sensation." You may not experience it, you may decide that it is too much to handle and wean, or you may ride it out and let your baby continue to nurse. We know of an older baby who was quite sensitive to his mother's feelings. As soon as she became uncomfortable she told him that her breast was "tired," and he matter-of-factly switched to the "fresh" breast. When the second side was also "tired," he was content to snuggle up to her and fall asleep without nursing.

• Eat a hearty, balanced diet and adhere to the pre-natal vitamin recommendations suggested by your medical professional. You need more rest than ever, which is difficult with a baby in the house. Daily naps when your baby naps are the best way to squeeze in extra rest. A new baby on the way need not cause you to deny your first baby any of the advantages of breastfeeding, provided you are in good health and take good care of yourself.

• If your older baby is still nursing by mid-pregnancy, you may want to think about nursing your older baby along with your new one—a procedure called tandem nursing. If you do not think you can accept this idea, try to gradually wean your older baby several months before the new one arrives, so your older baby will not remember nursing and feel displaced by the new baby.

If You Are Nursing Siblings (Tandem Nursing)

Tandem nursing is the term for nursing siblings who are not twins. Since it is quite possible to become pregnant while you are nursing a baby, you can continue nursing throughout your pregnancy and then nurse both the "old" baby and the "new" one.

How It Affects Nursing

• Most mothers report that tandem nursing is a delightful experience. It seems to alleviate some sibling rivalry: the "old" baby is not excluded and sees very clearly that he is loved as much as the "new" baby.

• Just as if you had twins, your milk supply will easily adapt to the demands of two babies.

What Can Be Done

• After the birth, there will be plenty of colostrum; for a few days the newborn should probably have "first rights" at the breast in order to receive his full complement of colostrum. After that it may not be necessary to feed the newborn first, although many mothers feel better about doing it. Many health-care advisors also feel strongly about always offering the breast to the new baby first.

• If you have an older baby who is eager to nurse, try to go home from the hospital as soon as possible. Doing so will minimize the effects of separation and enhance the bonding between the siblings.

• You might want to see that the older baby does not stake a claim to one breast; alternating sides is better for your supply and your newborn.

• Some mothers are ambivalent about nursing an older baby once the newborn has arrived. Mixed feelings, however, are natural and may be nature's way of preparing us for eventual weaning.

• Stay healthy by eating good, nutritious food and getting as much rest as possible; you will feel good and produce plenty of milk for your tandem nursers.

If You Have a Multiple Birth

Because multiples—twins and triplets—are often small babies, they particularly benefit from the nutritional advantages of breast milk.

How It Affects Nursing

• More than one baby will more than double the work required for their care, but the extra work and the problems are usually what one mother called "twin problems" and not "nursing problems." In fact, studies show that mothers of totally breastfed twins are more efficient and organized than mothers of supplemented or bottlefed twins.

• A mother of twins may be concerned about having an adequate supply of milk, but two hungry babies will stimulate enough milk to meet their demands.

• Some practical matters, like whether to nurse your babies

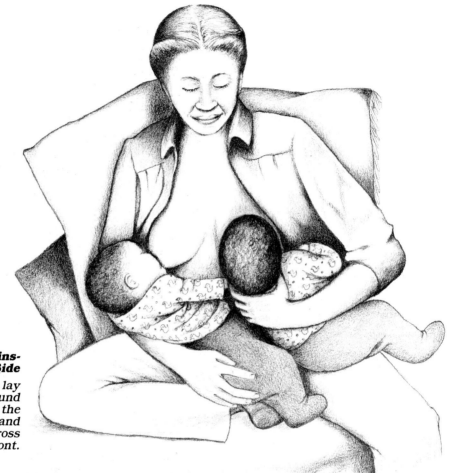

**Nursing Twins-
Legs To Side**

*A possibility is to lay
one or both around
your side in the
football hold, and
position other across
in front.*

separately or simultaneously, need extra attention at first, but
these concerns fade with experience.

**What Can Be
Done**

• Most breastfeeding mothers of twins find they easily have
enough milk for two, although some choose to supplement one
or both twins. Mothers of triplets usually find they need to
supplement, not necessarily because they cannot produce
enough milk, but because there simply are not enough hours
in the day to nurse all three babies.

• If you find yourself overtired from the demands of more than
one baby, take your babies to bed and nurse and snooze away
the afternoon.

• Make sure your diet is well balanced and your fluid intake
adequate. Many mothers find that a good vitamin supplement
helps them stay healthy and cope with stress.

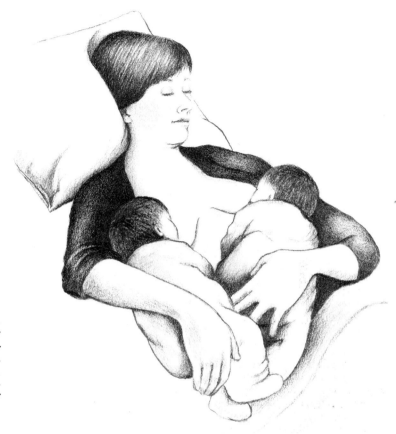

**Nursing Twins-
Legs Crossing**

*Try a variety of
nursing positions for
twins. Lay them in
your lap, crossing their
bodies close in front of
you.*

• A pressing dilemma for a new mother of twins is whether to feed her babies separately or simultaneously. Each method has its pros and cons, and only experience will help you decide which is better for you. Nursing them together saves time and tends to stimulate supply, but it is awkward, especially at first, and your babies may simply not be hungry at the same time. Nursing each separately allows special contact with each baby and is a little easier to learn. But you may end up feeling that you spend every waking minute with a baby at your breast, and there will be times when both are hungry at the same time.

• Try to avoid having one baby at the same breast all the time. Your baby misses out on the neurological advantages of dual-sided development gained by looking at his mother's face from both sides. (See page 14.)

• Mothers of breastfed twins are more prone to sore nipples, because it is more difficult to position two babies properly at the breast. Learning how to position properly and alternating feeding positions may help alleviate this problem. (See pages 46-48.) Encouraging each baby to suckle in a variety of positions at each breast also empties the breasts more thoroughly, decreases the likelihood of plugged ducts and boosts your supply.

• When you position your babies to nurse, remember that they are not fragile; in fact, they have just spent a crowded nine months together and love to be cuddled up next to one another! Try a variety of nursing positions: laying them extended out into your lap, crossing their bodies close in front of you, laying one or both around your side in the football hold, or any combination of these positions, as long as they are comfortable for the three of you. Use pillows or the arms of a chair as you need them.

• A great source of support is the newsletter, *Double Talk*, issued quarterly for parents of multiples.

If You Relactate or Have Lactation Induced

Relactation is the process of reinitiating the production of milk after prior lactation has ceased. It can take place days, weeks, months or even years after a prior breastfeeding experience. A similar but separate procedure is induced lactation, which involves establishing milk production in a woman who has never before nursed. Both processes are controversial today, even though they come from the days when wet nurses would relactate to save a baby whose mother had died. They are often viewed with disdain as unnatural or even rather perverted, although they are normal functions.

Relactation is an arduous task, requiring motivation, determination, patience, perseverance and understanding. A mother should never take lightly her decision to wean her baby with the thought that if she changes her mind, relactation will be simple. Any mother attempting induced lactation or relactation should seek out professional guidance and a good support system.

Why It Is Used There are four primary situations that call for induced lactation or relactation techniques.

1. When breastfeeding is delayed. A woman may choose to relactate after she or her baby has been ill or after an initial period of bottlefeeding.

2. After an untimely weaning. A woman may decide to relactate after a weaning caused by a medical concern, or she may simply change her mind after weaning.

3. When you adopt an infant. A woman may choose to induce lactation or relactate to feed an adopted infant.

4. To enhance normal lactation. A woman may find relactation techniques useful to enhance a diminished supply, such as after surgery.

How It Is Done   After weaning takes place, some of the alveoli and ducts are reabsorbed by the breast—a gradual process called mammary involution. Because of this involution, relactation is most successful if it takes place soon after the cessation of prior nursing. Induced lactation is a more difficult process, because during pregnancy the breast naturally prepares for lactation by developing more ducts and alveoli. A woman who has never been pregnant will have a less-developed mammary system.

The best stimulus for lactation is always breast and nipple stimulation, both sucking and massage. The mother can do a great deal of this, and often her partner finds emotional satisfaction as well as sexual pleasure in helping to prepare for a new adopted baby. However, if stimulation were the only factor, a lot of sexually active women would be producing milk when no baby was expected! Motivation and determination are also key factors affecting success.

Some drugs are available that tend to stimulate the process. Your health-care provider can help you evaluate them. There are also some mechanical aids available, the most common of which is the Lact-Aid Nursing Trainer®, a device that allows the baby to receive nourishment from a tiny tube along the nipple while simultaneously stimulating the breast to further production. Some relactating women also use breast pumps to stimulate their supply.

The fluid in a relactating breast will begin as drops of clear fluid that will turn blue or grey and eventually closely resemble mature milk. There is no colostral phase in relactation— colostrum is for newborns, and relactation is rarely for a brand new baby.

Relactation may affect your menstrual cycle or cause menstruation to cease as it does during lactation. Your menstrual cycle may also affect relactation; many women find that their supply decreases just prior to and during their menstrual flow.

A key question for a woman considering relactation or induced lactation is that of success. Is success defined in terms of productive lactation or in terms of a satisfying breastfeeding relationship for mother and baby? A mother who relactates may or may not be able to produce enough milk to feed her baby entirely from the breast. But most find tremendous joy and satisfaction in establishing that special relationship that breastfeeding affords while providing at least some of the baby's nourishment.

If You Are Traveling with a Breastfed Baby

Although traveling with a breastfed baby may cause you some concern, rest assured that it is much easier than traveling with a bottlefed baby. A little advance knowledge and planning will guarantee you an enjoyable and trouble free trip.

How It Affects Nursing

• Breastfeeding itself will have little or no effect on your trip. You may be in for some surprises if it is your first trip with a baby.

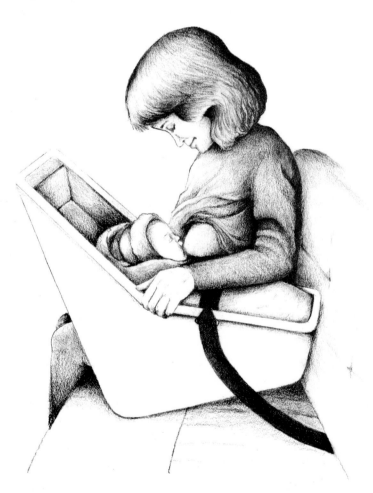

Breastfeeding In The Car

Some mothers find nursing in the car convenient. Buckle yourself into the seat beside your baby, who is in a rear-facing car seat. Lean over and across your baby to nurse while the car is in motion.

What Can Be Done

• Think about keeping things simple. Disposable diapers and baby wipes are easier than the cloth diapers and washcloths you may use at home. Although you may be tempted to dress your baby in adorable clothes to show him off, simple stretch suits are more comfortable and easier to launder.

• Plan your travel schedule with breastfeeding in mind.

By car. If you travel by car, plan many stops to nurse, play and stretch. Some mothers find nursing in the car is very convenient, but because it is not safe to drive with your baby out of the car seat, you really should stop the car each time your baby nurses. The question of convenience and practicality versus safety risk is yours to decide. One technique you might try is to buckle yourself into the seat beside your baby, who is strapped into a rear-facing car seat. If you lean over and across your baby, he will be able to safely nurse while the car is in motion. This may be inconvenient or even backbreaking, but it is worth a try.

By plane. If you travel by plane, keep your baby's sleep and nursing schedule in mind as you make your reservations. Many parents prefer to fly at night; not only do their babies sleep through the flight, but the fare is less as well! Nursing during take-off and landing helps to equalize the pressure in your baby's ears and makes him more comfortable.

When Breastfeeding May Not Be Possible

Although they are rare, some circumstances may make nursing impossible. Careful evaluation will help you and your health-care professional determine when breastfeeding may or may not be possible. Below are some guidelines to help. Notice that some items appear on each list.

Why Nursing May Not Be Possible

• A glandular problem in the mother

• Inappropriate prolactin levels

• Breast reduction surgery

• Some medical conditions, like a thyroid problem, Hepatitis B, extreme fever

• Some medications, like some thyroid medications, radioactive iodine, lithium

• A psychological aversion

When Nursing Is Possible

• A difficult or slow start

• A physically or mentally handicapped baby

141

• Breast reduction surgery

• Some medical conditions, like diabetes, tuberculosis, mumps

• Some medications, like types of penicillins, analgesics, antihistamines

• A reluctant mother

How Nursing Is Affected

While you may know in advance that you have a condition that precludes breastfeeding, nursing may also fail when you do not expect it to. Each of these circumstances is rare and different, but here are some signs that breastfeeding is not working. Do not abandon nursing too quickly if you notice only one of these signs; a combination of any two or more is a signal to look more carefully for an underlying problem.

• No breast enlargement during pregnancy.

• No perception of milk coming in within one to five days postpartum—no leaking, no fullness, no hardness.

• Baby seems to swallow little or not at all.

• Never see milk in or around baby's mouth.

• Few bowel movements, and fewer than six wet diapers a day.

• Baby does not regain birth weight by three weeks of age.

• Baby is unhappy. This one can fool you. Most mothers are overwhelmed by how demanding a new baby really is. Most new mothers think their baby is much unhappier than he should be.

What Can Be Done

• Get a good medical opinion from a medical professional who really supports breastfeeding. Unfortunately, many health-care professionals are still quick to recommend weaning when it may not be necessary. Get a second opinion if you are not satisfied. This is a standard practice in health care and shows good judgment, not mistrust.

• Find a support system. If breastfeeding does fail, you will most likely have to deal with frustration, anger and guilt.

• If breastfeeding really will not work, there are creative ways to use your breastfeeding skills and instincts to your baby's advantage.

1. Maybe you can continue partial breastfeeding and supplement with formula only the amount you cannot produce. Even if you are producing only a small amount of milk, you can offer your baby nurturing and comfort at the breast.

2. Many mothers continue every feeding at the breast, but use a Lact-Aid® to provide supplement.

3. You may feed your baby entirely by bottle, but use your breastfeeding skills: alternate feeding on left and right sides, hold and cuddle your baby throughout every feeding, get plenty of eye contact and practice demand feeding.

If you happen to be one of the extremely rare women who genuinely cannot produce enough milk, you need to feel validated that you did everything in your power to succeed at breastfeeding. You can give yourself credit for using your good mothering instincts and putting your baby's very real caloric needs before your very intense desire to continue breastfeeding at all costs. We hope that, rather than feeling defeated, you can come to terms with your problem and how unfair it is that it happened to you. Look to the compromises we offer above; they can help you make the best out of your situation. Your problem is truly insurmountable.

We hope that you will not encounter any health problem or difficulty that will lessen your breastfeeding experience. And statistics say that you probably will not. But should you be faced with any of the special circumstances described in this chapter, get the medical, practical and emotional help you need and remember that breastfeeding is one of the best gifts you can give your baby.

As Your Baby Grows Older

Starting Solids

As your baby grows older, well-meaning friends will frequently ask you when she is going to start eating real food. Although you are probably under the impression that breast milk is "real" food, you too may begin to wonder when you should offer your baby solid food.

The age at which babies start solid foods has often been determined by cultural standards and styles. We do have information, however, about the make-up of the infant that gives us important clues about the appropriate age for introducing solids.

Most babies are ready for solid foods between six and nine months, although an occasional baby is ready earlier. If, at six months, yours seems reluctant, do not force the issue; take the cue from her that she will be ready a little later. Most babies who refuse solids at six months are enthusiastic within the next few months, so try again every so often.

Why Wait Until Six Months?

• Before six months, a baby's digestive system may not be mature enough to handle foods other than breast milk. In addition, an immature digestive system does not really digest the food effectively enough for the baby to make use of the nutrients. Cereals, for example, are not good for infants under six months of age because young babies lack the enzyme necessary to digest starch. Some authorities think that forcing your baby's digestive system to operate beyond its capabilities can contribute to life-long stomach troubles.

• By starting solid food earlier than six months you replace breast milk in your baby's diet. Breast milk still provides the best and most usable nutrition for your baby. If she is filling up on the less nutritious solid foods, she may nurse less, you will have less milk and she will be missing her most important food source.

• Until she is about six months old, a baby has a tongue extrusion reflex—part of her nursing instinct—that prevents her from bringing food into the back of her mouth. An infant who is fed pureed baby food instinctively pushes it back out with her tongue and only swallows the smallest amount that slips through by accident. By six months of age, however, she can learn to coordinate the series of movements necessary to take in and swallow solid food.

• Beginning solids before six months can present the opportunity for many food allergies to develop. (See page 12.) In fact, you should delay introducing the more allergenic foods until after your child's first birthday. (See chart on page 149.)

• Evidence indicates that introducing solids before four to six months can lead to adult obesity. An infant needs about fifty calories per pound a day for the first year; solid foods simply add more calories to her diet than she can use. In addition, many parents tend to overfeed their children once they are on solid foods.

• At six months of age, your baby has the ability to sit up (probably with support) and hold her head up straight in a good position for eating. She also has the hand coordination necessary to reach for food and bring it to her mouth.

• By the middle of her first year, your baby's nutritional and caloric needs will increase, and she will demand more food and may seem dissatisfied after nursing. This is another clue for you that your baby needs some solid food in addition to breast milk.

• The iron supply your baby was born with will last for at least six months and then will begin to diminish; however, many babies have gone twelve months without solids and have not become anemic. Actually, anemia is rarely a breastfed baby's problem. Studies have shown that some common first foods like vegetables and fruits interfere with the absorption of iron from breast milk; pears, for example, cause a 76 percent inhibition of iron absorption. To prevent anemia, delay solids until your baby is old enough—again, around six months—to also consume iron-rich foods like meat and egg yolks.

Your baby does not need, and should not receive, iron supplements. The iron that is found naturally in your baby's food, combined with breast milk, will be more than adequate. Extra iron can interfere with the immunological action of lactoferrin in breast milk. (See page 10.) If, for some reason, you or your health professional suspect that your baby may be anemic and she has no interest in starting solids, your baby's blood can be tested. The results are usually reassuring, and you will not feel pressured to force solids on an unwilling baby.

The Role of Nursing in the Older Baby's Diet

Although many mothers expect that introducing solids will lead their babies to nurse less, this is rarely the case. Most breastfed babies continue to nurse as often as they did before starting solids. Their need for nursing has not diminished; they have just developed needs for additional foods.

Nutrition. The main thing to remember about your baby's nutrition during her first year is that breast milk is her most important food source. Although she needs to start solids sometime during the second half of her first year, they should be offered in addition to, not instead of, breast milk. Breast milk will supply a large percentage of her nutrition as a toddler, if she is still nursing at that age, and it continues to be your baby's best multiple vitamin.

Sucking Urge. Your baby still has a strong sucking need, and nursing still contributes to the development of her mouth and jaw. The need for sucking is so basic and so important that it should not be minimized in the interest of widening her culinary horizons.

Emotional Needs. The emotional significance of nursing is at a peak at this age. By six months your baby is alert and responsive, and she is in love with nursing. The love and security you communicate to her by nursing cannot be replaced.

How To Start Solid Foods

Starting solid foods is a step many parents look forward to eagerly. For one thing, it seems to be a landmark achievement in their baby's "growing up." Also, many parents anticipate the fun of offering new taste sensations to their child. As you start to offer your baby solid foods, pay attention to the general principles below.

• Be flexible. Babies, like adults, have food preferences. Your baby may seem to hate a certain food that is commonly given first. Do not struggle with it; just try something else. Your baby may also have clear opinions about wanting more or less than the recommended quantities. Listen to your baby. Forcing food is never a good idea, and it can lead to lifelong "eating

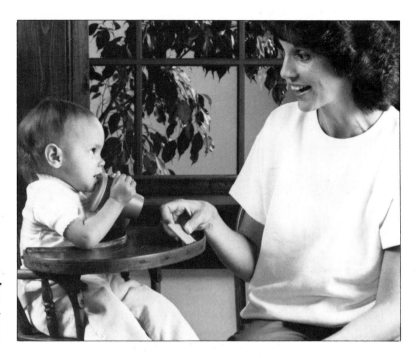

Introduction Of Solid Foods

Most babies are ready for solid foods between six and nine months.

problems." If your child is hungry, she will eat.

• Expect your baby to make a mess. At the age of six months, babies have very limited hand coordination. It is better for her to explore her food tactilely and thoroughly, than for everything to be neat and tidy. Have some washcloths handy.

• Feed your baby when she is in a happy frame of mind. It seems to work best to nurse the baby first, maybe on one side only, before offering solids.

• Give your baby food that is in as natural a state as possible. Avoid processed, packaged and canned food. Foods in their natural state are better for your baby, without the harmful additives you want to avoid and contain more of the nutrients you intend to offer your baby.

• Offer a new food by itself, not in combination with other foods, as in soup or a casserole. If your baby has an allergic reaction, you want to be able to pinpoint what caused it. After you introduce a new food, wait five days before introducing any other new item to her diet. This gives you a chance to observe your baby for a reaction (digestive, skin or other) and to feel sure that this food agrees with her. Avoid offering some foods (listed below) until your baby is a year old; some are likely to cause an allergic reaction and some offer other health risks.

Common Allergens— Wait Until Twelve Months

Citrus fruits and juices

Tomatoes

Egg whites

Milk and dairy products

Chocolate

Fish

Peanut butter

Foods to Delay for Safety

Honey—wait until twelve months to introduce honey, because raw honey can contain botulism bacteria.

Raw carrot sticks—do not give these to babies who have only front teeth. They can bite off a chunk that is large enough to cause choking.

Popcorn—avoid popcorn until your child can chew it.

Nuts—avoid because they can cause choking.

Foods to Avoid for as Long as Possible

Sugar

Carbonated beverages

Salt

Foods that contain additives

Condiments

Introducing Solid Food

Fruits and Vegetables. Your primary goal in introducing fruits and vegetables is to provide your baby with sources of vitamins A and C. You need to select foods with these vitamins, but remember that citrus fruits, because of their allergenic quality, should be delayed until your baby is a year old.

Foods Very High in Vitamin A

Apricots,

Cantaloupe

Carrots

Mangoes

Pumpkin

Spinach and other greens

Squash

Sweet potatoes

Foods Fairly High in Vitamin A

Apricot nectar

Asparagus

Broccoli

Nectarines

Purple plums

Foods Very High in Vitamin C

Broccoli

Brussels sprouts

Cabbage

Cauliflower

Cantaloupe

Grapefruit, grapefruit juice

Kohlrabi

Mangoes

Oranges, orange juice

Papayas

Peppers

Spinach

Strawberries

Foods Fairly High in Vitamin C

Asparagus

Bean sprouts, raw

Chard

Honeydew melon

Potatoes

Tangerines

Tomatoes, tomato juice

As your baby grows, add other fruits and vegetables that are in your diet as well. Your baby should soon adapt to eating what you eat at mealtime.

Breads and Cereals. Grains will add B vitamins, carbohydrates and bulk to your baby's diet. Crackers and bread (whole wheat toast cut into strips is a favorite) will supply grains. Do not overlook dry, unsweetened, unpreserved cereals, since they are good finger foods. Dry Cheerios are a sure winner with even the most finicky eater, and you can carry them in a small container in your purse and use them to quiet a restless baby.

If your family does not eat hot cereal, there is no reason your baby must have it. If you want your baby to have hot cereal, pass by the "baby cereals" in the supermarket. They are highly processed, not very nutritious, and have virtually no consistency. They are an unnecessary and expensive addition to your baby's diet. Give your baby regular oatmeal, a highly nutritious cereal, instead. If you want, you can put it through the blender or food processor to make it smoother. You can also offer Cream of Wheat, Cream of Rice, Malt-O-Meal or Familia, which are less processed than the "baby cereals." When you mix your baby's cereal, use expressed breast milk and no sweetener. You can also add some fruit for variety. In the beginning, avoid very coarse-grained cereals, like Wheatena, which are difficult to digest. Her diapers will look approximately like the bowl of cereal.

Protein Sources. You need to add iron and protein to your baby's diet, and meat, poultry, fish and eggs are good and common sources of both. The iron in meat is absorbed better than is the iron in vegetables.

Meat seems to be an acquired taste. Most babies do not like it at first, so you may have to disguise it. Chop it finely and then mix it with fruit or a sweet potato to make it more acceptable. Offering a chicken drumstick bone with a little meat on it is usually popular.

By the time your baby is receiving meat, you will have established her ability to handle many fruits and vegetables. So at this point a soup, stew or casserole might be an appropriate and tasty change for your baby. Other foods that contain protein include peanut butter (and other nut butters), yogurt and both hard and soft cheeses. These are also valuable additions to your baby's diet.

Some Cautions

• Avoid meat that contains nitrates and nitrites.

• Avoid fish that has come from contaminated waters.

• Offer your baby just the yolk of the egg, until she is one, because egg white is very allergenic. We know two popular ways to offer egg yolk: fry it into a small patty so it can be eaten by hand or take the yolk out of a hard boiled egg, mash it with breastmilk, and feed it to your baby with a spoon.

Offering Solid Food

• Keep the quantities small (about a tablespoon) in the beginning, and gradually build up to accommodate your baby's hunger and taste.

• Gradually include your baby in the family meals. As she takes more foods in greater quantities and uses her hands better, you can seat her in her high chair at the table with you at mealtime. Give her the same food you are eating if it is appropriate, but remember to take her portion out before you season the food.

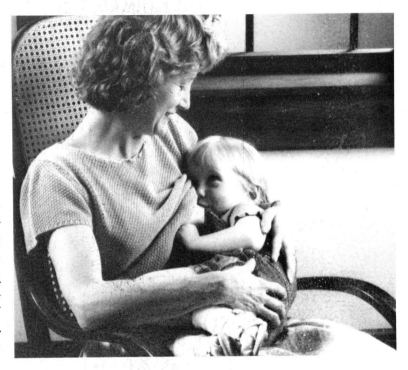

Breastfeeding An Older Child

The benefits of nursing an older child are significant: nutritional and immunological elements increase in concentration; nothing comforts an unhappy child the way breastfeeding can; and, it is a time for mother and child to share a cozy moment together.

• If you delay introducing solid food until she is six months old, she will progress fairly quickly from eating a little mashed food to eating chunks of finger food, virtually eliminating the need for buying baby food. While the baby food companies have taken the additives out of baby food, these foods are still more expensive than food you would make. And they are also often higher in calories than their homemade counterparts because they frequently contain starch.

• Buy a few small jars of baby food because they are convenient for taking along on an outing or a trip. They are also a convenient alternative for the baby if you have prepared something spicy like enchiladas or chili for the rest of your family.

Nursing an Older Baby

Before our babies are born, we all have notions about how long a baby should breastfeed, attitudes that come from our own parents, our friends, the media or other sources. But if, rather than looking to the culture for how long it can tolerate a nursing infant, we look at what infants do if they are left to nurse according to their own needs, we may get a very different picture.

In traditional societies, where breastfeeding takes its own course, it is typical that during the first year of life, the infant nurses continuously on and off throughout the day and night; during the second year, the baby gains mobility and begins to explore the world, but continues to nurse for both nourishment and comfort; between the ages of two and three, the baby develops much greater independence and gradually loses interest in nursing. She weans herself completely at some point during this period.

Some may find this pattern of breastfeeding quite acceptable while others may be put off by it. Nursing an older baby is certainly not mandatory and not all older babies need to be nursed. We do, however, want to offer reassurance that it is a healthy, natural, normal and beneficial practice.

And it can be a lot of fun. An older baby is a delight—she nurses with a definite sense of style. She may have favorite spots or positions (and they may even be a little out of the ordinary), and she will probably direct the whole affair. Her comical antics and acrobatics are usually a delight to her parents.

One more thought—nursing behaviors in your infant will become nursing habits in your toddler. You may or may not appreciate these habits. A baby may, for instance, twiddle the other nipple, twirl her mother's hair, or tug at her ear while she is nursing. These gestures of affection may not be annoying at first, but can become so. If you notice a nursing behavior that you do not want as a permanent part of your nursing relationship, discourage it from the start.

Benefits

Although the benefits of nursing an older child are not as well publicized as the benefits of breastfeeding a child during her first year of life, they are quite significant. While you will not often be encouraged to nurse your baby beyond the first year, you will be doing her many favors if you do.

• Studies of breast milk have revealed that, rather than diminishing, the immunological components actually increase with the age of the baby. In other words, as your baby begins to lose interest in nursing, your milk production system compensates for that and increases concentration of the nutritional and immunological elements your baby needs most.

• You can continue to offer nourishment and comfort to a sick or injured older baby. Nothing can comfort an unhappy child the way breastfeeding can.

• As always, breastfeeding provides an older baby with a great deal of emotional reassurance; such "refueling" is important for a baby who spends more and more time exploring the world.

Dealing With Criticism

Thanks in part to the recommendation of the American Academy of Pediatrics, nursing a baby through the first year has now won acceptance; in some circles, you may even find tolerance for nursing up to a year and a half. But if your baby is still nursing as she approaches two, you will sense disapproval from most of the people in your life. Some mothers and babies even nurse beyond the age of two, but you may not know about many of them; because of society's disapproval, they have discovered ways of making their nursing more subtle and discreet. If you do decide to nurse your baby beyond these boundaries, you will find it helpful to know how to deal with criticism.

• One way is to avoid the opportunity to receive criticism. Once your older baby is verbal, discuss the importance of nursing in private. Sometimes you can avoid nursing in front of those people who disapprove. Your baby does not need to hear the critical comments that people may make.

• Most people can accept the idea of late nursing better if they think you are in the process of terminating it. So tell people who are surprised to see that your baby is still nursing that, "She is weaning." What you are saying is true; she is weaning. Once your baby takes her first bite of solid food, she is in the process of weaning. Of course, for some babies this is a longer process than for others.

• If your nursing baby is old enough to talk, use a "special" word for nursing. Many babies use some baby-talk syllable to indicate that they want to nurse. Reinforce it; it may be very useful later. Just about anything except "breastfeed" or "nurse" will do, but the less understandable, the better. When you have company or are in the presence of people who will not be supportive of late nursing, your baby's demands to nurse will be disguised as general fussiness.

It may seem a shame to have to hide your lovely nursing relationship, but we all have special parts of other relationships that are private, too. Kissing and caressing your partner is healthy and normal, but most often done in private. You will feel better about your late nursing relationship if, instead of feeling odd or deceitful, you let it remain a healthy but private relationship.

Weaning

The whole issue of weaning, the process of discontinuing

breastfeeding, is controversial. You may be under pressure to wean sooner than either you or your baby is ready, or you may feel under another kind of pressure to nurse longer than you feel you want to.

Deciding when and how to wean (or when to let weaning take place) needs to be carefully considered. Both your needs and your baby's needs should be taken into consideration, of course, but be aware that at this age, your baby's needs are quite intense, and your decision to wean will have important ramifications. Before you plan a weaning date in advance, think about your baby and what weaning would mean to her.

During any weaning process, be sure to heap on extra attention and affection. It is important that your baby understands that you are not withdrawing your love. You are only making a transition with her. Since your baby associates nursing with your love, you do not want to plant any doubts in her mind as weaning takes place. Make a point to slow down during this time and focus attention and affection on your child in greater amounts than usual. This will help the weaning too, because your child will not be asking to nurse simply as a way of getting close to you. Fathers can also help the weaning process by increasing their involvement with their babies.

Below we present three philosophies and methods of weaning. You need to decide for yourself what feels right for you and take what you need from each philosophy.

Mother-Led Weaning

With mother-led weaning, the mother decides to wean her baby based primarily on her own needs and her desire to stop breastfeeding. A mother may wean for a variety of reasons. She may wean because she has a health problem requiring medication that will go through her milk and harm the baby. She may be going back to work and does not realize that she can continue to nurse her baby. She may wean because of a new pregnancy. Or she may simply not want to nurse any longer.

How To Wean

Whenever possible, plan a gradual weaning. It would be a mistake to wean a baby from the breast abruptly unless there was a genuine emergency. Sudden weaning would be emotionally traumatic for a baby, who would not understand the sudden withdrawal of such a basic and wonderful aspect of her existence. In addition, if you weaned your baby abruptly, you would become engorged and very uncomfortable. Unless you pumped your breast to cut back your milk production more gradually, you would probably get a breast infection as well.

Here are two methods of weaning a baby that avoid the problems associated with weaning too abruptly.

The Two-Week Method

We will base this description on the model of a baby who nurses six times a day. You may need to adjust this to match the actual number of feedings your baby has each day.

1. On the first two days, offer a bottle at one feeding and the breast at the other five.

2. On the third and fourth days, increase to two bottles and cut down to four nursings.

3. On the fifth and sixth days, offer three feedings from the bottle and three from the breast.

4. By the eighth and ninth days, decrease to two nursings and offer four bottles per day.

5. Between the ninth and the fourteenth day, cut down to only one breastfeeding per day and offer all the other feedings from the bottle. You can continue one nursing a day until you and your baby are ready to drop it.

The One-Month Method

1. Decide which nursing session your baby is least interested in. Substitute a bottle for that feeding each day for a week.

2. During the next week, substitute another bottle for the nursing you think would be the next easiest to give up.

3. In the third week, substitute another bottle for another nursing.

4. Continue this procedure until the last nursing has been eliminated.

This very gradual method has the advantage of allowing the baby to adjust and allows your milk production to diminish slowly.

Baby-Led Weaning

Baby-led weaning is simply the process of letting your baby nurse until she outgrows the need. She will gradually lose interest over a period of time and eventually stop nursing altogether. This process is often so gradual that you will not realize when your "last nursing" occurs.

Many mothers wonder when a baby would typically wean herself. The answer, as usual, depends on your baby's individual needs. It would be almost unheard of for a baby to wean herself before the age of one year. It would also be rare for a baby not to have weaned herself by the age of three.

The basic benefit of baby-led weaning is that it takes the guesswork out of this important developmental step. You do not need to agonize over whether this is the right time for your child to wean. You simply allow your baby to outgrow her need for nursing and gradually give it up, so you can feel confident that the needs that nursing satisfies are fulfilled.

If you choose this route, you will have to withstand a certain amount of pressure from many people in your life. But the respect you show for your baby's instincts will pay off in the confidence you feel about doing what is right for your baby. If you need more support and reassurance on the subject of baby-led weaning, read *Mothering Your Nursing Toddler*, by Norma Jane Baumgartner.

Mother-Guided Weaning

Mother-guided weaning is a variation of baby-led weaning. You pick up clues from your baby about her readiness to wean and then you gently and gradually introduce the idea to your child. This method is especially appropriate for a verbal baby who is nursing at a fairly late age, but shows no indication of weaning.

Occasionally toddlers do not seem to think of weaning on their own. Some are actually ready to wean, and nurse mostly out of habit. To suggest weaning to this type of child is actually giving her permission to wean. She may not have realized nursing was something to be outgrown, but will be receptive to the idea.

As you approach the idea of mother-guided weaning, keep this distinction between "needs" and "habits" in mind. A useful guideline is if a child is willing to give something up fairly easily and without much of a struggle (like a pacifier or a bedtime routine), it was a habit, but if she fights for it desperately, it is a genuine need. With this distinction in mind, you can evaluate your child's readiness to wean.

How does the mother decide if her child is ready to wean? She may take a clue from her child's age, although this is too arbitrary to be used as the only clue. If the child is between two and three, she will probably be receptive to weaning. If the child seems to nurse mostly when she is bored, take this as another clue. Your child may be happy to accept an alternative to nursing if one is offered.

How To Wean

1. Once you have decided that you think your child is ready, approach her with the idea of weaning. The first step is to discuss the concept that nursing is something we do when we are little, but as we get bigger, we can give it up. You can say that she may feel sad to think about not nursing anymore but there are many wonderful things that "big girls" and "big boys" get to do and that growing older is something to be looked forward to eagerly.

You might even tell a story (fictionalized, of course) about the time when you realized that you were old enough to stop nursing. You can add that you were a little sad about it, but that it was wonderful to get bigger and be able to play at a friend's house, ride bikes, climb trees or do whatever might sound big and fun to your child.

2. The next step is to set up a time framework for the weaning. Make it far enough in the future to allow plenty of time for discussing the idea over and over until she becomes comfortable with it. Many mothers successfully use an upcoming birthday as the weaning date. You can talk about it as the birthday approaches and help her to eagerly anticipate this milestone. Then, on her birthday, she can be easily distracted. (For example, when she comes in for her morning nursing, get up and open birthday presents instead. In all the excitement, she might easily forget the nursing.) You can also plot a weaning date out on the calendar or use an approaching season. Whatever you choose, make sure your child really understands what is being discussed.

Most importantly, remember that your basic assumption is that your child is ready to wean. If she resists, be flexible, accept your child's needs, and try again in a few months. When your child is truly ready, this method will work well and be a positive experience for both you and your baby.

As your baby grows older, you have challenges to meet as you attempt to satisfy her many needs and foster her growth. During this period of your child's development, the best advice you can get is: do not look to charts, books or averages for what you should do. Look to your child.

Chapter Ten

The Joys of Breastfeeding

N ow you know a great deal about breastfeeding, but facts and data about breastfeeding and its management, though exciting, are not the whole picture. Breastfeeding is much more than antibodies, convenience and good nutrition. Breastfeeding is joy, pride, satisfaction and love.

The women we have helped to breastfeed successfully have many common feelings that show this joyous side of breastfeeding. They appreciate the benefits, of course, but what really means the most to them are the intangible qualities associated with the entire breastfeeding relationship. We would like to share some of their thoughts with you.

Love

Breastfeeding mothers report a loving, intimate relationship with their babies that is so wonderful it is hard to describe. You can see it in their faces; they glow like teenagers in love for the first time when they speak of their babies. They ache to be with them again when they are apart for only a short time. They spend hours just watching their infants sleeping or nursing, and they long to be able to tell the world just how much love wells up in their hearts.

Shira tells of the mutual love she felt with each of her breastfeeding sons:

"How often putting one of my babies to the breast reminded me of how precious life's moments can be— taking time to give warmth, nurturing, caring and a sense of well-being and then receiving unconditional love and trust in return. Gurgling and slurping, exploring my neck, nose, ears and shoulders with his chubby hand, or pulling his face away momentarily to check out the wider world and then coming right back—each of my babies quickly and endearingly learned how to keep me close to him.

"The memory of each one's sweet breath, warm, soft skin, and twinkling gaze still brings me delicious feelings I can reach out and relive. Having the opportunity to nurse both boys made me genuinely feel that whatever sensory and growth experiences they gained from our breastfeeding time together, at every stage I reaped my full reward, too."

Breastfeeding, for Shira, was a true loving relationship, a two-way street, with both mother and baby feeling love, feeling loved and feeling lovable. Breastfeeding is the honeymoon phase of your relationship with this brand new person, and you are sure to be amazed at the quality and purity of the love you feel.

Intimacy

The dearest part of most loving relationships is the intimacy, defined as "private, closely personal," and not necessarily sexual. Each relationship is different, but when there is intimacy, there is deep satisfaction in the privacy of the relationship. The lovers know each other in a way no one ever has or ever will.

All breastfeeding mothers find that an intimate relationship develops between them and their babies. Their gazes, caresses and shared joy become the language of their love, known only to them. Fathers, too, develop their own private relationships with their breastfeeding babies. As a breastfed baby delights in his warm relationship with his mother, he becomes irresistably lovable. So his father pours out his love, and a new circle begins.

As Connie describes some of the loving aspects of her relationship with her son, Ian, you can sense the joy she receives from knowing him in a way that no one else does:

"Sometimes I think my darling son, Ian, is simply continuing to nurse as a courtesy to me. I am a sensual person, and he knows how much I enjoy snuggling up with him after a hectic day—just the two of us as one contented unit. He knows how I love those quiet early morning nursings in bed when his hand skims softly over my belly. He knows how hilarious I find his antics with my breast when he's in a jolly mood, kneading it with great relish or letting go with an audible pop to look around and giggle.

"Nursing has been the most delightful experience of my

life, my secret joy. In the early months I enjoyed knowing I was sustaining his life with my body, but now that our nursing relationship is almost strictly for comfort, I enjoy it even more. I have seen him grow from a squalling infant to a happy, independent toddler. I know he still needs me when I see his nursing increase dramatically during his sick times or when he practically leaps into my arms to nurse before bed after gleefully escaping from me after his bath and rocketing naked around the room."

Your breastfeeding relationship will be an intimate one, fulfilling and satisfying. You will enjoy the confidence of really knowing your baby and understanding his needs. But mostly you will have that "private, closely personal" relationship that is exclusively yours to enjoy.

Satisfaction

It is one thing to know the value of breastfeeding, but another thing entirely to experience it firsthand. Many mothers look at the decision to breastfeed in the same way they look at deciding to take vitamins each day. There is clearly value in taking vitamins, and you will feel better about yourself knowing that you are doing a "good" thing.

But that is where the comparison ends. Breastfeeding is one of the rare cases where doing the right thing is also pleasurable.

As Mary relates a bit of her breastfeeding experience, you see that she knows in her head the good things that breastfeeding means. But she goes on to describe the fulfillment that comes when the knowledge becomes anchored; what she knew to be right, she comes to feel in her heart:

"Most of us breastfeeding mothers can appreciate only secondhand the more practical benefits of breastfeeding. We do not really know what it means not to provide our children with that invaluable colostrum or to have an infant who is constipated from the wrong formula. We have never experienced the nuisance and extra work of making formula and fussing with bottles, and trying to warm a 2 a.m. night feeding for a frantically hungry baby. We have never had to take a trip with a car trunk full of the paraphernalia necessary to feed a baby on the road. In some ways, we don't really appreciate how wonderful breastfeeding is.

"But there is one practical side of breastfeeding that I can come very close to thoroughly appreciating—how reliably it comforts my sick or hurting child. Having heard my son, Michael, cry in terror of some night fear, moan in pain from a high fever, call out for comfort when his poor little body is banged or bruised from his ever-constant attempt to conquer the world, or waken in the middle of the night, frantic with the irritation of his newly budding teeth cutting through raw, sore gums, I can readily know what it would be like to have no immediate source of comfort for him. And nothing during these times has ever worked better or faster than nursing. I pick up my crying child, hold him to my breast, and hear his eager sucking between fast-fading sobs. As I watch his last tears (for now) leave the corners of his eyes, he finds in me some ease from his trouble."

This satisfaction, so comforting to any nursing pair, is especially valuable to a mother who is employed and regularly separated from her baby. Marion enjoys the benefits of breastfeeding for her babies' health, as well as for the satisfying feelings she receives from doing the best for them:

"Breastfeeding became increasingly important to me after I returned to work when my daughter was about two months old. It gave me a quiet time at the end of the day that I could look forward to sharing with her, and it made me feel that I was offering her something very special. That helped, particularly on the days when I got 'the guilts' about leaving her at the sitter's when I went to work.

"In addition to providing psychological benefits to both of us, I believe that nursing protected her physical health. I never missed a day of work because she was ill while I was nursing, and I am convinced that it was due to the immunities my milk provided. I am now nursing my second child and working, and I believe that breastfeeding has contributed immeasurably to my having two healthy, secure children. And I still look forward to the satisfaction of coming home and nursing my baby."

We not only enjoy the satisfaction of breastfeeding, we absolutely delight in it. Connie relates her pleasure in nursing her baby and we feel her joy, too:

"The greatest joy I find in nursing is the same as what we experience when we see someone digging enthusiastically into a solid meal, or when I see my two little boys in the tub on their stomachs kicking away in unison like two giddy tadpoles. It is the joy of watching children do what they do best, have a genuinely good time!"

Although breastfeeding is indeed delightful, we experience many more rewarding emotions as well. Having a new baby at home can be taxing and frustrating, but breastfeeding offers comfort, confidence and security as successful elements. A classic story is Michele's:

"After long months of waiting, my daughter was born, pink and beautiful and healthy. Immediately after her birth I put her to my breast; she nursed avidly. My mothering experience at this point was wonderful. I felt so successful, nourishing and loving my baby in the same simple act.

"Eventually the time came for diaper and clothes changes. Emily was working to adjust to her new environment (even breathing was new to her) as I fumbled with maladjusted diaper tapes and the extremely complex system of snaps on a sleeper. Inevitably we both would become frustrated with these more practical, and difficult, aspects of our new relationship. Thankfully, we could always quickly and simply return to the bastion of success and comfort we discovered after only moments of acquaintance—baby nursing.

"This association with ease and relaxation continued even as the more practical parts of our day became simpler. After playing and laughing or a bump on the head, nursing provided for both of us a feeling of peacefulness and comfort.

"Emily, at one year, is every day exploring the world further away from my lap. In time, she will return there only for hugs and kisses. When she is grown, I am certain our nursing experience will seem to have been very brief. Therefore, we are both relishing this special time we now share. I cannot help but think that our nursing relationship is fostering a strong lifelong bond."

Obviously, Michele's nursing relationship is good not because Emily received colostrum and will have fewer allergies, but because both Emily and Michele enjoy the ease of success, the peace and the whole of their relationship.

Many of us start out thinking it would be wise to breastfeed our babies, and the incredibly enjoyable aspects of breastfeeding reaffirm in us our desire to do so. What a marvelous gift— we do a good thing and are reinforced by its pleasure!

Emergence of Motherhood

But beyond the satisfaction, beyond the intimacy and even beyond the love, there are some intangible qualities to breastfeeding that are unlike any other experience a woman will ever know.

A woman goes through a giant phase of psychological growth

in the short span of a breastfeeding relationship. She begins feeling pride and satisfaction in her decision to nurse, and that feeling grows into her intimate relationship with her baby. Through that relationship, she feels more connected to her baby, to herself as a child, to herself as a mother, to her mother and to all mothers. Step by step, she experiences growth in her personal life, her relationship with her baby, her motherhood and her womanhood.

As this growth process begins to take place, most women find themselves taken by surprise. Dana tells of her expectations, but listen to her sweet surprise as she discovered that the reality is far better than her expectation:

> "I knew that when my baby was born I would nurse him. I had read enough to know that breastfeeding was the best choice I could make. And I was eager to feel like a mother—to devote myself entirely to the care and attention I knew he would need. I just could not wait to have my baby and grow to love him.

> "But I was taken by absolute surprise, the sweetest of my life, when not only did I love him more than I thought possible, but he responded and loved me too. I knew he would be the center of my universe for at least a time, but found myself reveling in the fact that I was clearly the center of his universe as well. He obviously loved me as intensely as I loved him. I just did not expect a tiny baby to be like that."

This surprising delight is the springboard for the emergence of motherhood. We do not usually have expectations of how motherhood will actually feel, so when we experience firsthand how wonderful it really is, we are encouraged to grow more as mothers. We find, to our amazement, that we have strong feelings of motherliness and protectiveness. We feel the deep urge to see that our baby is happy, healthy and protected.

We gradually come to see motherhood as an entity in itself, not just our particular state at the time. And we finally experience the connecting point in the cycle of our female sexuality. For many mothers, like Debra, there is great pride and satisfaction in the growth and development a woman experiences through motherhood:

> "The greatest thing about nursing is mostly how proud it makes me feel of myself (and my husband, because he supported me), that we somehow managed to do it the best way for our daughter. To nurse from birth on through a course of baby-led weaning in toddlerhood is a tremendous accomplishment for a woman, and certainly out of

the ordinary today. So many of us do not realize how lactation is just that next step in our chain of sexuality, and it is important to complete that cycle.

"I have always wondered what it was about the way my parents raised me that allowed me to view my pregnancy, birth and breastfeeding with the attitude I did—trusting in my body and how it is supposed to work—and complete my cycle with incredible enjoyment. Within this cycle, pregnancy, birth and breastfeeding have been important experiences for me. What I am basically trying to say is that my self-esteem has been greatly enhanced. I feel very proud of myself and confident in the wisdom of my choices."

Just as motherhood enhances womanhood, breastfeeding enhances motherhood. Breastfeeding helped Debra feel pride in her motherhood, and feeling good about motherhood evolved into feeling pride in her womanhood.

A woman who has experienced this type of growth knows her value, feels satisfaction in her efforts and appreciates herself as a woman. Through breastfeeding, many mothers find this growth and satisfaction. They discover that they love breastfeeding, they love being a mother and they love being a woman.

Conclusion

During the years we have spent teaching women about breastfeeding, we have been asked countless times, "If breastfeeding is so natural, why do I need to learn how to do it?"

Although breastfeeding is indeed natural, breastfeeding knowledge is not instinctive. Rather, it is a learned behavior which is passed down socially. In *Breastfeeding in Practice*, Elizabeth Helsing and F. Savage-King share this delightful knowledge: "Suckling of the young is learned rather than instinctive behavior in many other mammals too. For example, when an elephant has her first calf, experienced cows surround her and guide her to feed it. Dolphins behave in a similar way."

In the past, knowledge about breastfeeding was passed down informally from one generation of women to the next. Much was learned by the constant example of the visible nursing mothers, and some extra information was also transmitted verbally as "common knowledge."

This chain of knowledge was broken during the bottlefeeding era that peaked during the fifties and sixties. As younger women grew up, they no longer had a source of information about breastfeeding, so the few who tried to nurse looked to the medical profession for help. But since breastfeeding was not and is not a major topic of study in medical schools, little help was available. It became more and more difficult to find the help and support needed to learn to breastfeed successfully.

Even today, many women have never actually seen a baby nursing at the breast until their own baby is brought to them for the first feeding. No wonder we so often see breastfeeding mismanaged and ended early.

Since we do not have mothers and aunts with breastfeeding knowledge and advice to offer us, today we must look to the growing body of knowledge that is coming from other women of our generation who have successfully breastfed their babies. In addition, we are fortunate that the recent increased popularity of breastfeeding has caused study and research on the subject to proliferate.

This book is an attempt to combine both of these important sources of breastfeeding knowledge into a practical, readable and, most of all, usable guide. We hope that, for you, this will be the link that joins you to the chain of breastfeeding knowledge that mothers are recreating today.

Resources
Breastfeeding

Books

The Breastfeeding Guide for the Working Woman (Wallaby Books/Simon & Schuster), by Anne Price and Nancy Bamford. Offers the information a woman needs if she wishes to continue breastfeeding after returning to work. Covers some basic breastfeeding information plus "how tos" on pumping, storing, and transporting breast milk. Also includes suggestions for making arrangements at your work place to facilitate breastfeeding.

The Womanly Art of Breastfeeding (Plume), by La Leche League. LLL's official manual. Contains excellent breastfeeding information, plus personal anecdotes and support for the woman who chooses to be a full-time mother.

Mothering Multiples (LLL), by Karen Gromada, R.N. Full of practical tips for nursing and mothering twins and triplets. Can be purchased at local La Leche League groups, or ordered from LLL. Write to the Order Dept., LLLI, 9616 Minneapolis, Franklin Park, IL 60131.

Mothering Your Nursing Toddler (LLLI), by Norma Jane Baumgartner. If you are nursing a toddler, or will be, this book offers information and support for the joys of continued nursing.

Equipment

• *Breast Shields (for inverted nipples). Order from La Leche League at the above address.*

• *The Happy Family Breast Milking and Feeding Unit. It can be ordered from Happy Family Products, Inc., 12300 Venice Blvd., Dept. CE, Los Angeles, CA 90066.*

• *The regular Lact-Aid Nurser Trainer® and the deluxe set, which contains a larger number of the supplies, can be ordered from Lact-Aid International, Inc., P.O. Box 1066, Athens, TN 37303.*

• *Comfy-Dry Nursing Pads (reusable) can be ordered from Happy Family Products, Inc., 12300 Venice Blvd., Dept. CE, Los Angeles, CA 90066.*

• *If you need an electric pump, the Axi-Care company has a wide range to choose from. Write them for information Axi-Care Pumps, Neonatal Corporation, One Blue Hill Plaza, Pearl River, NY 10965.*

Drugs and Breastfeeding

Books

Drugs in Breast Milk (ADIS Press), by John T. Wilson. The most comprehensive overview on the subject of drugs in breast milk. Contains information on the factors affecting the transmission of drugs into milk, but provides no table of drugs. Geared more toward the clinician or researcher.

Pamphlets

"Breastfeeding and Drugs in Human Milk," by Gregory J. White, M.D., and Mary Kerwin White, (LLL publication #505). A 48-page booklet that lists drugs, whether they go through to breast milk, and what their possbile effects on the nursling would be. Also provides medical references. Can be ordered from the La Leche League.

"Drugs in Breastmilk: A Consumer's Guide," by Paula C. Rothermel, B.S., and Myron M. Faber, M.D. A ten-page pamphlet that lists drugs by categories and whether they go through milk and the possible effect on the nursling; also provides medical references. Can be ordered from the Birth and Life Bookstore, P.O. Box 70625, Seattle, WA 98107.

Organizations

La Leche League International, 9616 Minneapolis, Franklin Park, IL 60131

Parenting

Books

Pregnancy, Childbirth and the Newborn (Meadowbrook Press), by Penny Simkin, R.P.T.; Janet Whalley, R.N., B.S.N. and Ann Keppler, R.N., M.N., of the Childbirth Education Association of Seattle. A complete guide for expectant parents. This authoritative, easy-to-use and thorough book can be ordered from the distributor Simon and Schuster, 1230 Avenue of the Americas, New York, New York 10020.

Right from the Start (Rodale), by Gail Sforza Brewer and Janice Presser Greene. The authors contend that an informed parent is more able to meet the challenges of motherhood. Then they lay out good information (with charts and checklists) about care of your unborn and newborn baby.

Self-Esteem for Tots to Teens (Meadowbrook Press), by Eugene Anderson, Ed.D., George Redman, Ph.D., and Charlotte Rogers, Ph.D. Shows how to use five easily remembered principles to build your child's self-esteem. Can be ordered from the distributor Simon and Schuster, 1230 Avenue of the Americas, New York, New York 10020, order number 0-671-54467-5.

Your Child's Self-Esteem (Doubleday), by Dorothy Corkille Briggs. In this book you will learn not only the theory behind developing good self esteem for your child and its importance, but also the practical methods for making sure it happens.

Touching: The Human Significance of Skin (Harper and Row), by Ashley Montagu. Montagu explores the importance of the skin as a sense organ, the role of touch in our physical and emotional lives. He focuses on infancy and has information on the importance of breastfeeding. This book is a favorite of ours.

The Family Bed (LLLI), by Tine Thevinin. The author examines the history of family sleeping and its benefits, and she dispells some myths about this practice. It is very supportive to parents who want to keep their children in bed with them.

How to Really Love Your Child (Victor Books), by Ross Campbell, M.D. The premise of this book is that most parents truly love their children, but many children do not feel that love. The author offers specific and concrete methods for making sure your children feel your love.

Crying Baby, Sleepless Nights (Warner Books), by Sandy Jones. The author explores the possible physical causes of infant crying and sleeplessness. In addition she discusses your baby's basic needs, the issues of crying and sleep, and strategies for parent survival.

First-Year Baby Care (Meadowbrook Press), edited by Paula Kelly, M.D. A step-by-step guide to almost every aspect of caring for an infant, this book also offers information on safety, infant development, and medical care. Can be ordered from Simon and Schuster, 1230 Avenue of the Americas, New York, New York 10020. Order number 0-671-54579-5.

Newsletters

Mothering Magazine. Addresses all aspects of mothering. You can find articles on family health, mothering, fathering, the child's world, mid-wifery, alternative education, nutrition and more. It can be ordered from Mothering Magazine, P.O. Box 2208, Albuquerque, NM 87103.

Double Talk. A quarterly newsletter for parents of multiples. It offers articles, features, interviews and book reviews for parents of twins or triplets. It can be ordered from Double Talk, P.O. Box 412, Amelia, Ohio 45102.

Equipment

• The McPack is an excellent choice for an infant frontpack. Your baby can face either toward or away from you, and can fit in the pack for up to two years. This pack has extra seat and head support and a comfortable strap design. It allows you to reach in and touch your baby while he is in the pack. It can be ordered from McPack, 9552 W. Capri, Littleton, CO 80123.

Organizations

The Couple to Couple League International, Inc. (family planning) P.O. Box 11084, Cincinnati, OH 45211

Health Care

Books

The Ms. Guide to a Woman's Health (Anchor/Doubleday), by Cynthia W. Cooke, M.D., and Susan Dworkin. The information in this book is extremely thorough. It is very consumerist and stresses the importance of a woman's participation in her own health care. The book explains many medical terms and procedures, and these explanations will help you to better assess your doctor's recommendations. It emphasizes throughout that you need to take responsibility for making your own decisions.

Our Bodies, Ourselves (Touchstone/Simon & Schuster), by The Boston Women's Health Book Collective. By now this book could be called the classic woman's health care guide. It is a very complete and excellent reference for any woman's health-related issue.

Pamphlets and Newsletters

"Relief From Backache During Pregnancy and Breastfeeding" by Georgann Marx, D.C., and Anne Price. This excellent pamphlet by a chiropractor outlines the type of back strengthening a woman can do to prepare for pregnancy. It also includes exercises and information for optimal back comfort during pregnancy. In addtion, there is a section specifically designed to alleviate the type of back pain a new breastfeeding mother might experience. It can be ordered from Back Support Press, 2993 S. Peoria, Suite G-9, Aurora, Co 80014.

"The People's Doctor," by Robert Mendelsohn. M.D. Dr. Mendelsohn offers an alternative view on a different medical subject in each issue and cites research to substantiate his claims. His basic approach is noninterventional and his opinions are often unorthodox. This newsletter is informative. Each issue includes a column by Marion Thompson, former president of La Leche League. This monthly newsletter can be ordered from The People's Doctor: A Medical Newsletter for Consumers, P. O. Box 982, Evanston, IL 60204.

Nutrition

Books

Nourishing Your Unborn Child (Avon), by Phyllis S. Williams. You will find a total guide to pre-natal nutrition in this book. It has specific information on your nutritional requirements during pregnancy, what to avoid, diet for the post-partum period, plus menus and recipes.

What Every Pregnant Woman Should Know: The Truth about Diet and Drugs in Pregnancy (Random House), by Gail Sforza Brewer and Tom Brewer. This is truly what every pregnant woman should know—the clear facts about prenatal nutrition, with menus and recipes.

Supermarket Handbook (Plume), by Nikki and David Goldbeck. This handbook is a thorough guide to the foods we find in the supermarket. You will learn how to get the most nutrition for your dollar, the meaning of food labeling, and some nutritional guidelines.

Laurel's Kitchen (Bantam), by Laurel Robertson, Carol Flinders, and Bronwen Godfrey. A vegetarian cookbook and more. It is an excellent and interesting source of nutritional information, and the recipes are delicious. In addition is the fascinating account of who "Laurel" is, which sets the tone for this special book.

Pamphlets

"As You Eat, So Your Baby Grows," by Nikki Goldbeck. This pamphlet offers specific information on pre-natal nutrition. It is excellent and accessible information. It can be ordered from Ceres Press, P.O. Box 87, Department D, Woodstock, NY 12498.

Bibliography

Applebaum, R. M., M.D. (1979) "Management of lactation problems" *Symposium on Human Lactation* p. 69

Beske, E. J. and Garvis, M. S. (1982) "Important factors in breastfeeding success" MCN 7:174-79

Bing, Elisabeth and Colman, Libby (1977) *Making Love During Pregnancy* Bantam Books, NY

Bhaskaram, P. and Reddy, V. (1981) "Bactericidal activity of human milk leukocytes" *Acta Paediatrica Scand* 70:87-90

Brewer, Gail Sforza and Greene, Janice Presser (1981) *Right From the Start* Rodale, PA

Brewer, Patricia (1979) *You Can Breastfeed Your Baby....Even in Special Circumstances* Rodale, PA

Chan, G. M. et al. (1982) "Growth and bone mineralization of normal breast-fed infants and the effects of lactation on maternal bone mineral status" *AM. J. CLIN. NUTR.* 36: 438-43

Coffin, Lewis (1974) *The Grandmother Conspiracy Exposed: Good Nutrition For The Growing Child* Capra Press, CA

Committee on Drugs (1983) "The transfer of drugs and other chemicals into human breast milk" *Pediatrics* Am. Acad. of Pedr.

Countryman, Betty Ann, R.N., M.N. (1978) "Breastfeeding and Jaundice" LLLI Info. Sheet no. 10

Countryman, Sandy (1980) "Breastfeeding Your Premature Baby" LLLI Info. Sheet no. 13

Dahms, Beverly Barrett, M.D.; Kraus, Alfred N., M.D.; Gartner, Lawrence M., M.D.; Klain, David B., M.D.; Soodalter, Jane, B.A.; and Auld, Peter, A.M.,M.D. (1973) "Breastfeeding and serum bilirubin values during the first four days of life" *Jour. Of Ped.* 83: 1049-1054

De Carvalho, Manoel, M.D.; Hall, Michael; and Harvey, David (1981) "Effects of water supplementation on physiological jaundice in breast-fed babies" *Arch Dis Child* 56:568-69

De Carvalho, Manoel, M.D.; Klaus, Marshall, M.D.; Merkatz, Ruth B., R.N., M.S.N. (1982) "Frequency of breastfeeding and serum bilirubin concentration" *Am J Dis Child* vol. 136

Ewy, Donna and Roger (1975, 1983) *Preparation For Breastfeeding* Signet, NY

Frantz, Kittie B., R.N., CPNP (1980) "Ineffective suckling as frequent cause of failure to thrive in the totally breastfed infant" *Human Milk: Its Biological and Social Value*

Frantz, Kittie B., R.N., CPNP (1980) "Techniques for successfully managing nipple problems and the reluctant nurser in the early postpartum period" *Human Milk: Its Biological and Social Value*

Gartner, Lawrence M., M.D. (1979) "Breastfeeding and jaundice" *Symposium On Human Lactation*

Gartner, Lawrence M., M.D. (1983) "Hospital policies, breastfeeding and neonatal jaundice" *Breastfeeding Abstracts* vol. 2 no. 4

Garza, C. et al. (1983) "Changes in the composition of human milk during gradual weaning" *Am Journ. of Clin Nutr* 37:61-65

Gerrard, John W., M.D.; and Shenassa, Mehdi, M.D. (1983) "Food allergy: two common types as seen in breast and formula fed babies" *Annals of Alergy* vol. 50 no. 6

Goldman, A. S. et al. (1983) "Immunologic components in human milk during weaning" *Acta Pqaediatr Scand* 72:133-34

Good, Judy (1980) "Breastfeeding the Down's Syndrome Baby" LLLI Info. Sheet no. 51

Grady, Edith (1980) "Breastfeeding the Baby with a Cleft of the Soft Palate" LLLI Info. Sheet no. 82

Gross, S. J. et al. (1980) "Nutritional composition of milk produced by mothers delivering pre-term" *Jour Pediatrics* 4:641-644$_2$

Gruskay, F. L. (1982) "Comparison of breast, cow and soy feedings in the prevention of onset of allergic disease" *Clin. Pediatr.* 21:486-91

Gutherie, Richard A., M.D. (1983) "Jaundice" *A Practical Guide to Breastfeeding* the C.V. Mosby Company p. 200-210

Helsing, Elisabeth with Savage-King, F. (1982) *Breast-Feeding In Practice* Oxford University Press, New York, Toronto

Hull, V. J. (1981) "The effects of hormonal contraceptives on lactation: current findings, methodological considerations, and future priorities" *Studies In Family Planning* 12(4) 134-155

Hymes, James (1974) *The Child Under Six* Prentice-Hall, NJ

Jarranpaa, A. L. et al. (1982) "Milk protein quantity and quality in the term infant I. metabolic responses and effects of growth" *Pediatrics* 70: 214-20

Jelliffe, Patrice E. F., M.P.H., F.R.S.H. (1979) "Nutritional Aspects of Human Lactation" *Symposium On Human Lactation* p. 25

Kramer, M. S. (1981) "Do breastfeeding and delayed introduction of solid food protect against subsequent obesity" *Jour. Ped* 98:883-87

La Leche League International (1981) *The Womanly Art of Breastfeeding* LLLI, IL

La Cerva, Victor, M.D. (1981) *Breastfeeding: A Manual For Health Professionals* Medical Examination publishing Co., Inc., NY

Lawrence, Ruth A. (1980) *Breastfeeding: A Guide For The Medical Profession* The C. V. Mosby Company, St. Louis, Toronto, London

Lemburg, Patti (1979) "Nursing my Twins" LLLI Info. Sheet no. 54-a

Lemons, J. A. et al. (1982) "Difference in the composition of preterm and term milk during early lactation" *Pediatr. Res.* 16:113-17

Lunn, et al. (1980) "Influence of maternal diet on plasma prolactin levels during lactation" *Lancet* 8169:23-25

Maisels, M. J. et al. (1983) "Breastfeeding, weight loss and jaundice" *Journ. Of Ped.* 102:117-18

Marano, Hara (1979) "Breastfeeding: New Evidence It's Far More Than Nutrition" *Medical World News* vol.20 no. 3

Marx, Georgann, chiropractor, and Price, Anne (1984) "Relief from Backache During Pregnancy, and Breastfeeding Care During Pregnancy and Breastfeeding" Back Support Press

Messenger, Marie (1982) *The Breastfeeding Book* Van Nostrand Reinhold Co., NY

Montagu, Ashley (1971) *Touching: The Human Significance Of The Skin* Columbia University Press, NY and London

Newton, Niles, Ph.D. (1979) "Key issues in human lactation" *Symposium On Human Lactation* p.25

Nicoll, Angus; Ginsburg, Robert; and Tripp, John H. (1982) "Supplementary feeding and jaundice in newborns" *Acta Pediatr Scand* 71:759-761

Ojofeitimi, E. O. (1982) "Effect of duration and frequency of breastfeeding on postpartum amenorrhea" *Pediatrics* 69:164-8

Oski, F. A. and Landaw, F. L. (1980) "Inhibition of iron absorption from human milk by baby food" *Am Jour Dis Child* 134:459-60

Poland, R. L. (1981) "Breast milk jaundice" *Jour. Pediatr* 99:86-87

Prema, K. and Phillips, F. S. (1980) "Lactational amenorrhea—a survey" *Indian J Med Res* 71:538-46

Price, Anne and Bamford, Nancy (1983) *The Breastfeeding Guide For The Working Woman* Wallaby Books/Simon & Schuster, NY

Pryor, Karen (1963,1973) *Nursing Your Baby* Pocket Books, NY

Rothermel, Paula C., B.S. and Faber, Myron M., M.D. (1977) "Drugs in Breastmilk—A Consumer's Guide" *Birth And The Family Journal* vol.2:3

Ribble, Margaret (1943, 1965) *Rights Of Infants* Signet, NY

Riordan, Jan (1983) *A Practical Guide To Breastfeeding* The C. V. Mosby Company, St. Louis, Toronto, London

Saarinen, U. M. (1982) "Prolonged breastfeeding as prophylaxis for otitis media" *Acta Paediatr. Scand.* 71:567-71

Satter, Ellen, R.D. (1983) *Child Of Mind: Feeding With Love And Good Sense* Bull Publishing Co., CA

Sirigatti, Susan Z., editor (1983) "Human Milk An International Newsletter" *DJ* Colgate Medical Ltd., NY

Slaven, Sylvia and Harvey, David (1981) "Unlimited suckling time improves breastfeeding" *Lancet* 1:392-93

Stanway, Penny and Andrew (1978) *Breast Is Best* American Baby Books, WI

Wharton, B. A. (1982) "Food for the suckling: revolution and development" *Acta Paediatr. Scand. Supp.* 299 p.5-9

White, Gregory J., M.D. and White, Mary Kerwin (1980) "Breastfeeding and Drugs in Human Milk" *Veterinary And Human Toxicology* vol. 22, suppl 1

White, Gregory J., M.D. and White, Mary (1982) "Medications for the Nursing Mother" LLLI Info. Sheet no. 21

White, Mary (1973) "Diarrhea in Infancy" LLLI Info. Sheet no. 15

Whitehead, R. G.; Paul, Allison A.; and Cole, T. J. (1982) "How much breast milk do babies need?" *Acta Paediatr. Scand. Suppl.* 299 p. 43-49

Yaffe, Sumner J., M.D. and Waletsky, Lucy R., M.D. (1979) "Drugs and chemicals in breast milk *Symposium On Human Lactation*

Index

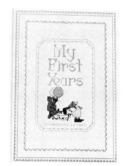

My First Years

A beautiful baby record book to save your precious memories from arrival day to kindergarten! The colorful padded cover is reproduced from an original cross-stitch design of the *My First Friends* animals, with a delicate framing border. There are 32 pages of popular subjects like the family tree, a growth record, medical history, the first birthday, favorite photos, and many more. It is also gift boxed to be the perfect shower or new-arrival gift.

(S & S Ordering #: 54543-4) $10.95

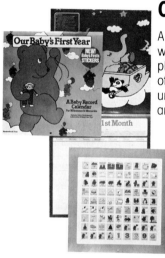

Our Baby's First Year

A colorful spiralbound baby record Calendar that hangs on the nursery wall for handy use! OUR BABY'S FIRST YEAR is a "universal date" calendar plus a record book: 13 complete months for recording the "big events" of baby's first year as they happen. The day-by-day write-in spaces are undated, so OUR BABY'S FIRST YEAR starts whenever the baby arrives and lasts 13 months—a complete first year!

Each month features a colorful baby animal nursery character to decorate the room, plus month-by-month development and baby care tips for quick reference. There's even a family tree and birth record form! A colorful and practical baby gift!

(S & S Ordering #: 54486-1) $7.95

Parents' Guide To Baby & Child Medical Care

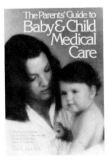

A first aid and home treatment guide that shows parents how to handle over 150 common childhood illnesses in step-by-step illustrated treatment format. Edited by Terril H. Hart, M.D., it contains: — *index of symptoms — record forms — height and weight charts — accident prevention — childproofing tips.*

(S & S Ordering #: 54470-5) $7.95

"If you have a new baby, you need this book. It is really the most useful baby medical guide available."

—Mitch Einzig, M.D.
Children's Health Center,
Minneapolis, MN

Parenting Books

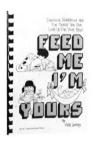

Feed Me! I'm Yours
by Vicki Lansky

America's most popular baby food and tot cookbook. Over 200 recipes and ideas for easy and economical ways to make baby food and for sneaking nutrition into infants, toddlers and tots. Practical, gifty, spiral-bound edition — *Corn off the Cob Hot Cereal — M&M Cookies — Egg Posies — Simpler Souffle — Valentine Crispies — Bunny Biscuits — plus milk-free cooking, travel food recipes, kitchen crafts and more.*

(S & S Ordering #: 54480-2) $6.95

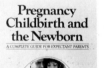

Pregnancy, Childbirth, and the Newborn
by the Childbirth Education Assn. of Seattle

Developed by one of the oldest CEA groups in the country, this book is the most complete up-to-date illustrated guide to pregnancy and childbirth available. It offers expectant parents a comprehensive and objective guide to all the options available to them.

(S & S Ordering #: 54498-5) $9.95

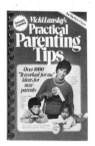

Practical Parenting Tips
by Vicki Lansky

Over 1,000 parent-tested ideas for baby and child care that you won't find in Dr. Spock's books. Vicki's newest bestseller is the most helpful collection of new, down-to-earth ideas from new parents ever published. Practical ideas for saving time, trouble and money on such topics as: — *new baby care — car travel — toilet training — dressing kids for less — discipline — self-esteem.*

(S & S Ordering #: 54487-X) $6.95

Dear Babysitter
by Vicki Lansky

Peace of mind at least! For new parents who finally get to go out to a movie again, here's a way to make sure the kids *and* the sitter are safe and happy. Really *two* ways: DEAR BABYSITTER includes a 48-page Sitter's Handbook of basic first aid and emergency procedures, games and activity suggestions for all age levels up to 7, techniques for enforcing your "house rules", and bedtime strategies.

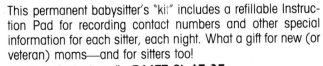

This permanent babysitter's "kit" includes a refillable Instruction Pad for recording contact numbers and other special information for each sitter, each night. What a gift for new (or veteran) moms—and for sitters too!

(S & S Ordering #: 54477-2) $7.95

Special Gift Books

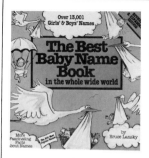

The Best Baby Name Book In The Whole Wide World

America's best-selliong baby name book by Burce and Vicki Lansky. More names, more up-to-date, more helpful, more entertaining, more gifty than any other baby name book! — *over 10,000 boys' and girls' names . . . more than any other book — how to name your baby: 15 rules — name psychology and stereotypes.*

(S & S Ordering #: 54463-2) $3.95

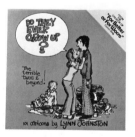

Free Stuff For Kids

Over 250 of the best free and up-to-a-dollar things kids can get by mail: *— badges & buttons — games, kits & puzzles — coins, bills & stamps — bumper stickers & decals — coloring & comic books — posters & maps — seeds & rocks.* FREE STUFF FOR KIDS is America's No. 1 best-selling book for children!

(S & S Ordering #: 54468-3) $3.50

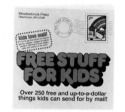

Hi Mom! Hi Dad!

101 cartoons about all the funny things that happen after you get your baby home, during the first twelve months of parenthood. It's a great remedy for post-partum blues.

(S & S Ordering #: 54482-9) $3.95

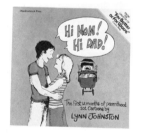

Do They Ever Grow Up?

A hilarious, 101-cartoon survival guide for parents of the tantrum and pacifer set. It's all about the terrible two's and the pre-school years. Lynn Johnston's funniest book yet!

(S & S Ordering #: 54478-0) $3.95

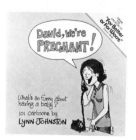

David, We're Pregnant

101 laughing-out-loud cartoons by Lynn Johnston that accentuate the humorous side of conceiving, expecting and giving birth. It turns all the little worries of pregnancy into laughter.

(S & S Ordering #: 54476-4) $3.95

ORDER FORM

_____	54476-4	David, We're Pregnant!	$ 3.95
_____	54482-9	Hi Mom! Hi Dad!	$ 3.95
_____	54478-0	Do They Ever Grow Up?	$ 3.95
_____	54486-1	Our Baby's First Year	$ 7.95
_____	54470-5	Parents' Guide to Baby & Child Medical Care	$ 7.95
_____	54477-2	Dear Babysitter	$ 7.95
_____	54543-4	My First Years	$10.95
_____	54487-X	Practical Parenting Tips	$ 6.95
_____	54480-2	Feed Me! I'm Yours!	$ 6.95
_____	54498-5	Pregnancy, Childbirth, and the Newborn	$ 9.95
_____	54463-2	Best Baby Name Book	$ 3.95
_____	54468-3	Free Stuff for Kids	$ 3.50

Simon & Schuster, Inc.
Simon & Schuster Building
1230 Avenue of the Americas
Dept. MBA
New York, NY 10020

Please send me copies of the books checked above. I am enclosing $_____ (full amount per each copy and $1.00 to cover postage and handling).

Send check or money order payable to Simon & Schuster. No cash or C.O.D.s please. For purchase over $10.00, you may use VISA/MasterCard; card number, expiration date, and customer's signature must be included. Allow up to six weeks for delivery.

☐ MasterCard   ☐ Visa

Credit card # _____

Expiration date _____

Signature_____

Name _____

Address _____

City_____ State_____ Zip_____